Rethinking experiences
of childhood cancer

Rethinking experiences of childhood cancer

A multidisciplinary approach to chronic childhood illness

Mary Dixon-Woods, Bridget Young and David Heney

Open University Press

Open University Press
McGraw-Hill Education
McGraw-Hill House
Shoppenhangers Road
Maidenhead
Berkshire
England
SL6 2QL

email: enquiries@openup.co.uk
world wide web: www.openup.co.uk

and Two Penn Plaza, New York, NY 10121–2289, USA

First published 2005

A catalogue record of this book is available from the British Library

ISBN–13 978 0335 21255 2 (pb) 978 0335 21256 9 (hb)
ISBN–10 0 335 21255 7 (pb) 0 335 21256 5 (hb)

Library of Congress Cataloguing-in-Publication Data
CIP data applied for

Typeset by YHT Ltd, London
Printed in the UK by Bell & Bain Ltd, Glasgow

The *initial blood test* oil painting by Susan Macfarlane is part of a national touring
exhibition *Living with Leukaemia* promoted by the charity *A Picture of Health*.

Acknowledgements

Shona Agarwal provided invaluable assistance in literature searches, managing the bibliographic database and preparing the manuscript. Dr Emma Ross helped with literature reviews and drafts of chapters containing medical information and we gratefully acknowledge her help. We would like to thank all the patients, families and staff of LRI Ward 27 for their unfailing support over the years.

This book is dedicated to Bill, Miriam, Colin, Jonny, Anne, Veronica and Ruth.

Contents

1 Approaches to childhood and childhood cancer

In this book we aim to show how the study of experiences of childhood cancer can benefit from a multidisciplinary approach that recognizes the contribution of the range of social sciences, and that is informed by a sound understanding of the clinical issues in the diagnosis and management of childhood cancer. There are important reasons for revisiting the social science study of childhood cancer at the present time. First, a well-founded social science perspective on childhood cancer is necessary not only for researchers, but also to inform policy and practice in relation to the care of children with cancer and their families. However, some of the most important contributions to the field (for example, Bluebond-Langner's classic study of the private world of dying children, published in 1978) were written during a period when childhood cancer had poor outcomes, and a majority of children died of the disease. Though many of Bluebond-Langner's insights still hold about the ways in which strict social codes governing social interaction about childhood cancer evolve, it is no longer the case that most children with cancer die. For example, survival for children with leukaemia has improved dramatically, with more than three-quarters of children now surviving. Childhood cancer remains an important threat to life – it is the second leading cause of death in children, exceeded only by accidents – but issues of living with cancer and survival are of increasing interest and form the key focus of this book.

Second, the social science study of childhood in general is burgeoning (James et al. 1998; Jenks 1996a; Lee 2001; Mayall 2002), with the emergence since the mid-1980s of a 'new' sociology of childhood. This has taken the route of distinguishing how a sociology of childhood might differ from a psychology of childhood, and it has been successful in identifying previously ignored questions and encouraging the application of methods consistent with those questions. With the development of the wider field of childhood studies, there are opportunities for refreshing and deepening our understanding of experiences of childhood cancer.

At the same time, social science exploration of a specific serious childhood illness exposes some of the problems in applying the concepts and arguments of the 'new' social studies of childhood to serious childhood illness. To date, while there has been growing interest in the social science, and particularly the sociological study of child health (for example, Mayall 1998), the absence of a sociology of childhood *illness* has been striking, especially given the enormous progress of the sociology of illness applied to adults. Study of childhood cancer specifically has tended to be dominated by quantitative psychological approaches. We argue that psychological approaches have much to offer and have an important place, but we offer a critique of how they have been used thus far in childhood cancer. We emphasize that the potential offered by more interpretive approaches, and use of a more diverse range of research strategies and theoretical approaches, has yet to be fully exploited. We hope to demonstrate the need for a more fully developed sociology of childhood illness as well as the need for caution about rejecting the contribution of other disciplines from the field of study.

Third, there is now a substantial body of empirical research on experiences of childhood cancer. Though the quality of this work is variable, it is important to begin to synthesize it so as to produce an integrated and holistic account of the evidence, to identify where the gaps might lie, and, something we will emphasize throughout this book, to identify an agenda and directions for future research. It is also appropriate to synthesize the work on childhood cancer with empirical and theoretical work in other fields. For example, the sociology of adult illness has much to offer in terms of a theoretical approach to experiences of serious chronic disease, particularly in the absence of a more fully elaborated sociology of childhood illness.

We begin in this chapter by outlining briefly the 'new' social studies of childhood, and then offer a preliminary critique of this as it applies to the study of experiences of childhood cancer. We suggest that any social science approach to childhood cancer must be firmly grounded in an understanding of the clinical issues, and we offer a summary. We conclude by proposing that experiences of childhood must be studied in ways that explicitly reject rigid disciplinary boundaries, and recognize that an understanding of experiences of childhood illness involves an understanding of familial contexts and, crucially, of parenting.

The 'new' social studies of childhood

It has been argued that sociology has traditionally excluded children as objects of attention, tending to leave them to the psychologists, and considering them of interest only in so far as they are the objects of socializing processes (James et al. 1998), or studying them only indirectly though subdisciplinary areas of education, gender and the family, rather than studying them as a topic in their own right (Brannen and O'Brien 1995). A new sociology of childhood can be dated to around the late 1980s, when a body of theoretical and empirical work began self-consciously to carve out what later came to be known as the new social studies of childhood, although the beginnings of much of the critique that forms its core can be traced back to earlier work (Aries

1962; Denzin 1977). Taken together (though there are various positions within the body of work, and increasing evidence of diversity), the literature in the new social studies of childhood has a number of distinct features:

- a challenge to what are perceived to be the dominant accounts of childhood;
- a focus on the social construction of childhood;
- a focus on children's agency (their ability to act on the world) and the implications of this;
- an interest in the ways that children are oppressed by the ways in which they are socially constructed.

A challenge to the 'dominant account' of childhood

Central to the new social studies of childhood is a critique of the 'dominant framework' (Lee 2001) within which, it is argued, children and childhood are currently conceptualized. This framework consists of discourses – organized and distinctive ways of thinking and talking about specific issues – that privilege particular views of children and childhood. These have consequences for our understandings of the ontology (concerned with how things are) of childhood, and have normative consequences (concerned with how things should be) for children's power and status.

'Dominant framework' discourses are identified within the new social studies of childhood as being founded on developmental understandings of childhood, which model childhood as a progression towards becoming more thoroughly adult (Qvortrup et al. 1994). These discourses construct children as 'becoming' human and adult, not as 'being' human and adult. The dominant account is seen to be heavily influenced by those working in the tradition of Jean Piaget, who proposed a series of predetermined stages through which children must progress in order to achieve rationality. James et al. (1998) mount a direct challenge to this approach, which they see as constructing childhood as a 'natural' state, (too) directly connecting biological with social development. Developmental psychology is further identified as the source of a highly influential and pervasive discourse that results in children being seen as immature, irrational, incompetent, asocial and acultural. Those working within the new social studies of childhood have criticized the account of childhood offered by developmental psychology as being only one of many possible accounts, as being empirically unsustainable, and as having unpalatable political (and other) consequences for children (Mayall 2002). They call attention to the other possible accounts of childhood, arguing that many of these (particularly those rooted in a view of the diversity of childhood and of children's agency) are more legitimate and have more positive implications.

The social construction of childhood

Much of the new social studies of childhood turn on the idea that childhood is not simply (or solely) a biologically constructed category: it is a socially constructed state. Social constructionism, as an approach, calls into question the taken-for-granted nature of social phenomena, and sees the social world as the product of the ways in which people give meaning to the world through their actions and interactions (Stainton Rogers and Stainton Rogers 1992). Such an approach argues that childhood is neither a self-evident 'fact', nor a descriptor of a naturally occurring biological phrase. Instead, 'childhood' is a particular cultural phrasing of the early part of the life course, is historically and politically contingent and subject to change (James and James 2001a) and the common-sense assumptions that underlie childhood are themselves objects of study. A key project within the new social studies of childhood, then, is to explain and deconstruct the discourses that have established taken-for- granted 'truths' about childhood (James et al. 1998).

According to this position, childhood is, therefore, emphatically not a universal state with stable features, and images of what a child can be, is, or should be are generated socially (Moss et al. 2000). Some have argued, for example, that the qualities deemed 'natural' to childhood, including 'innocence' and 'vulnerability', have varied over time and in different cultures (James and Prout 1990). Others have gone as far as arguing that childhood itself is a relatively modern invention (Aries 1962). Adolescence, as a particular variant of childhood, has come in for similar treatment. Lesko (1996, 2001) offers a critique of the supposedly distinctive nature of adolescence, arguing that myths about young people being controlled by their hormones, peer-oriented, and a source of threat, are historically and socially specific phenomena, but have led to particular forms of practices (especially practices of control) in relation to young people. Discourses around childhood, then, are strongly linked to practices and policies, and become in Moss et al.'s (2000) terms a 'regime of truth'.

> Foucault calls such conventions – our ways of naming things and talking about them – *discourses*, and those discourses that can exercise a decisive influence on a specific practice can, in his view, be seen as 'dominant discursive regimes' or 'regimes of truth'. Such regimes serve a disciplinary or regulatory function: they order or organise our everyday experience of the world, influencing our thoughts, ideas, and actions.
>
> (Moss et al. 2000: 236)

The argument that children (among whom, for the sake of elegance of expression and as a heuristic device, we include young people) belong to a socially and culturally constructed category that we know as 'childhood' has a number of implications. First, it implies that the 'universal child', proceeding through a series of predetermined stages posited by Piagetian developmental psychologists, is a myth. Instead of a single universal child, there are many different childhoods, constructed through many different discourses, including the discourses of children themselves, in many different contexts. James et al. (1998), therefore, emphasize the diversity of childhood, and call for the deconstruction of childhood's 'conventional, singular and reductive form', enjoining us to stop thinking of 'the child' and to think instead of children, and how children experience 'childhood'.

Second, proposing that 'childhood' is a social category (not simply a chronological, biological, or developmental category), opens it up for sociological attention. The new recognition that childhood is socially produced and negotiated within specific social relations means that while we understand biological maturity as a fact, we recognize that, like gender and ethnicity, biology is not the sole determinant of the social state.

The absence of children from the sociological agenda until the 1980s has been attributed to the implicit assumption that children are adults in the making. Oakley (1994) and Brannen and O'Brien (1995) note the absence of research on (or with) children, even within topics such as education, that directly relate to their interests and concerns. They suggest that this neglect was due to an interest in the forces of socialization – how children become incorporated as members of society – and how these contributed to the bigger questions of class and equality (Pole et al. 1999). The processes of socialization were, then, of more interest than children themselves. The emphasis was not on what children are, but on what they are not: their value in becoming, not in their being. Recent work has seen a sustained attempt to avoid seeing children simply as the passive pawns of socializing processes, and has instead constructed them as having agency – the ability to act upon the world (for example, Alanen and Mayall 2001).[1]

Third, social constructions embodying assumptions about the needs and competences of children are made evident in law and social policy as well as in the everyday interactions that adults have with children (James and James 2001a). These have considerable implications for children's rights and experiences. For example, it is argued that developmental psychology has specified the parameters of 'normality' in childhood, promoting particular ideas of what children are or normally should be (Stainton Rogers and Stainton Rogers 1992). These ideas then inform social and health policies in relation to children, and result in particular forms of practices. Similarly, most dominant accounts treat the idea of children's 'vulnerability' as self-evident, and although vulnerability can be shown not to be as linear or clear as is often assumed (Frankenberg et al. 2000), it strongly affects social interactions between children and adults, policy and practices.

Children as social agents

Central to the manifesto of the new social studies of childhood is an attempt to position children as active social agents. Children are thus ontologically rehabilitated, and rescued from 'presociological' (James et al. 1998) understandings that construct them as passive. It is of course necessary to find some means of explaining how it is that children *do* come to participate in social life. Most accounts (self-consciously avoiding the term 'socialization') fall back on some form of structuration theory (Giddens 1984), which tries to reconcile human agency (the ways in which people act on the social world) and social structure (the ways in which people are constrained by the social world). These accounts point out the need to address both the extent to which children are influenced through external forces (structure), and the extent to which they can shape their own understandings and behaviour (agency) at the same time.

> Children are and must be seen as active in the construction and determination of their own social lives, and the lives of those around them and the societies in which they live. Children are not just passive subjects of social structures and processes.
>
> (Prout and James 1997: 8)

In their later work, James and James (2001a) simplify this axiom by proposing that: 'childhood not only shapes children's experiences, but children also help shape the nature of the childhood that they experience' (p. 30). The North American sociologist Corsaro (1997) adopts a similar position, describing what he calls 'interpretive reproduction' as an alternative to the focus within psychology on the *individual child's* development and adaptation to society. Interpretive reproduction aims to capture the idea that children do not simply internalize society and culture, but actively contribute to cultural production and change. It also implies that children are, by their very participation in society, constrained by the existing social structure and by society reproduction. Corsaro's formulation can be seen as a helpful attempt to understand how it is that children become incorporated in society, but are also agents of change and sustenance within society. His analysis is, of course, closely allied to Giddens's work, and it provides a useful approach to many aspects of childhood, including the production of peer cultures. It also demonstrates, in its focus on how children are constrained by social opportunity structures, links with Bourdieu's theorization of social life (Bourdieu 1990). Corsaro, interestingly, also accepts that the ways in which children construct the world are different from those of adults, arguing that a sociology of childhood must recognize developmental changes throughout childhood as well as variability in these. This is a concession that appears to be have been made relatively recently (and relatively grudgingly) by others working in the new social studies of childhood.

Children as a disadvantaged group

Perhaps unsurprisingly, an interest in the cultural politics of childhood is a defining feature of the new social studies of childhood (James and James 2004). The key unifying themes of this work have concerned the inappropriate construction of the ontology of children by the 'dominant accounts' of childhood, which has resulted in a number of unfortunate consequences for children, the positioning of children relative to the dominant adult group and the implications of their minority status for their ability to be taken seriously. This dimension of the new social studies is important, as it does not stop at identifying the social constructions of childhood, but attempts to move beyond this and reconstruct childhood in what is believed to be a more favourable way.

Within the general field there are a number of different positions and extremes of position in adopting a radical agenda, which we shall return to in more detail in Chapter 7. At one extreme the children's liberation movement of the 1970s (for example, Holt 1975) describes childhood as a form of slavery. More commonly, a 'minority group' model has been identified (James et al. 1998) as one of the major ways in which children are theorized within contemporary sociology. In this model, children are characterized as a marginalized group, discriminated against by oppressive adults. Mayall (2002) explicitly argues for a politicized sociology of childhood, stating that: 'I regard children as a minority social group, whose wrongs need righting.'

Some have drawn parallels between the disadvantaged status of children and the disadvantaged state of other socially constructed categories. Oakley (1994) for example, explicitly links a child emancipation agenda with a feminist agenda, proposing that children and women share the characteristic that they are both members of minority social groups, deprived of rights, and both 'hidden in the ideological apparatus of "the family"'. Indeed Butler (1996) argues that the evolution of feminist sociology, in the process of elevating the status of women's work in domestic labour, increased the tendency to objectify children by treating them as the objects of mothering. One of their early projects of the new sociology of childhood, therefore, was to 'rescue' the study of children from the sociology of the family, where, according to James and Prout (1996), they were seen but not heard within traditional sociology. Mayall (1994b, 2000), and Oakley (1994), for example, seek to liberate children from being conceptualized as subsumed within families: 'We must extricate children, conceptually, from parents, the family and professionals' (Mayall 2000: 243).

The discursive treatment of children as essentially 'incompetent' (Hutchby and Moran-Ellis 1998a), or 'vulnerable' (Christensen 2000), is seen as key to how childhood comes to be subject to oppressive practices. 'Dominant' accounts of childhood are criticized for promoting these qualities as being natural and inherent to childhood, in particular because dominant discourses are prone to becoming incorporated into professional practices and regulatory regimes (Moss et al. 2000), informing and reflecting social economic policies towards children and the institutions that manage them (Stainton Rogers and Stainton Rogers 1992). In this way the view that children are incompetent, irrational, vulnerable, and require protection (Mayall 1996) comes to be institutionalized.

Children are then deemed to be incapable of exercising important rights, including rights of participation in decisions concerning their own bodies, and are prevented from having influence on powerful institutions of society, for example by being denied a vote, excluded from consultation, and open to interference and surveillance at every level. Their construction as incompetent means that their ability to act as moral or political agents is undermined in favour of an approach that seeks to protect and control them and emphasizes their dependence on adults (Storrie 1997). Dominant discourses strengthen their claim to control children's lives by specifying what is normal, proper and good about childhood, so that educationalists, social workers and others can claim expertise in monitoring, categorizing, and managing childhood and children (Scott et al. 1998). Mayall (2000) for example, identifies children as a subordinated group (like women), and comments that children and childhood have become the object of massive interventions, with whole armies of health and social workers working to modify childhood based on concepts of children's needs that derive from professional assumptions, priorities and goals. Jenks (1996a) similarly argues that children find their daily lives shaped by statutes regulating the pacing and placing of their experience.

At the same time, it is argued, children are marginalized and prevented by adults from participating in decisions that affect them, through oppressive practices which are themselves founded on these inappropriate conceptualizations of childhood (Roche 1999). By failing to recognize children's *ontological* agency, therefore, dominant accounts also lead to children being denied *political* and *moral* agency. It is also suggested that this effect is demonstrated in, and reinforced by, a neglect of children as a subject of study in their own right, and an adult-centred approach to research that has left unheard the voices of children themselves. Qvortrup (1997), for example, argues that children are hidden in the statistical accounting of the state, counted as 'dependants' and excluded as a unit of reference.

An effort to challenge the marginalization of children is taken on as a political task by the new social studies of childhood. A key task is to offer an alternative account (or accounts) of childhood, that is more valid, legitimate and authentic and has more positive consequences for children. This includes, in particular, an attempt to challenge the understanding of children as (inevitably) incompetent and irrational by locating 'developmental' constructions of 'the child' as a politically, historically and culturally specific understanding (James and Prout 1990), not an inevitable consequence of childhood itself (Lansdown 1994).

A social science approach to childhood cancer

It is clear that the social science study of childhood is developing rapidly. However, while we have seen interesting developments in the sociology of child health (for example, Christensen 2004; Mayall 1996), an emerging sociology of the body as it applies to childhood (Prout 2000), and a number of promising individual studies, we have not yet seen the development of a fully elaborated sociology of childhood illness. Many of the tenets of the new social studies of childhood provide an important framework within which to explore and understand experiences of serious childhood illness and will inform our analysis in this book as well as the agenda we draw up for future research. The need for a phenomenological approach that investigates the perspectives of those affected by childhood cancer, and the need to construct children as having agency and being active in the creation of meaning, are central to this. However, we also want to draw attention to some potentially problematic aspects of the new social studies of childhood in attempting to understand the experiences of childhood cancer.

In particular, we suggest that there are some key flaws in its identification of children as a social group, its tendency to deny aspects of childhood that might have a developmental or biological basis, its failure to adequately locate children within families or to recognize the role that parents play in co-producing their children's health or their own experiences of their children's illness, and its exclusion of the contribution of psychological theory and methods. We also argue that the normative and ideological aspirations of some of the liberationist positions adopted within the new social studies have important implications that have not yet been fully explored either empirically or theoretically.

Childhood cancer and the social construction of childhood

Qvortrup's (1994) repositioning of the child as an active social agent, together with Brannen and O'Brien's (1996b) insistence that children be studied by sociologists as beings in their own right (psychologists have been doing this for years), are clearly hugely important in terms of establishing children as subjects of social science study. This position characterizes children as interacting and engaging with people, institutions and ideologies to forge a place for themselves in social worlds, and who, by demonstrating the interactive properties of a social agent, are worthy of inclusion and study alongside adult individuals and social groups. These arguments help to restore to children some of the reflexivity and agency denied them in traditional social science study, particularly, as we shall see later in this book, in research on childhood cancer. Throughout this book we will theorize children and young people as active, interpretive agents and as 'beings' in their own right.

However, we do not necessarily subscribe to all of the consequences which many of those working within the new social studies of childhood argue to follow from this position. An obvious set of criticisms concerns those which apply to any social constructionist analysis of a field (Bury 1986), including the potential for a descent into relativism (Wyness 2000), in which no one form of knowledge is seen to be more valid than another. As Pole et al. (1999) identify, the notion of childhood being something created through discourse (i.e. though talking about it) may neglect the more straightforward 'realities' that underlie childhood.

A related problem with social constructionism is that it tends to avoid identifying what affects most children and the common features of childhood (Wyness 2000). This manifests in important ways, for example, in the tendency to reject social constructions of children as vulnerable and incompetent as having any validity. Recent work on children's views of health has indeed begun to show the relevance and value of seeking their understandings, and much of the work done in this vein has focused on showing how assumptions about children being invariably incompetent are flawed. However, as we show in our chapter on children's involvement in decision making (Chapter 7), the *nature* of children's competence needs to be properly understood, and there is a danger that perceptions of children's general competence may be taken as normative prescriptions about children's participation in decision making. From identifying that vulnerability or incompetence are social constructions, some of those working within the new social studies of childhood then move to assuming that children are *not* vulnerable and that they should be assumed to be competent (for example, Alderson 1993a; Mayall 2002), and so given rights of decision making. This move from theoretical position to normative prescription makes for a number of difficulties in relation to childhood cancer.

Linked to this, we suggest that the identification of children as a distinct social group, and the attempt to claim for them a radical agenda of rights, is part of an attempt to impose the status of victimhood for children. As Holstein and Miller (1990) suggest, 'victim' is a categorization device that provides a set of instructions for understanding social relations, and also functions as a rhetorical device that encourages partisan activity intended to persuade others to adopt and act on preferred understandings of people and circumstances. Constructing childhood and adulthood as being locked in a victim/oppressor relationship (as they have been in some of the writing in the new social studies of childhood) is, we suggest, inappropriate and unsympathetic. It is a static and partial vision of relations between children and adults that neglects the ways in which power is negotiated and situated. Moreover, no sustainable account is offered in the new social studies of childhood of how people move from one state (victim) to another, more despised state (oppressor).

There are also important problems with the characterization of children as a social group, particularly when efforts are then made to find commonalities between children and other disadvantaged social groups, such as women (Oakley 1994). An obvious conceptual problem is that, unlike traits such as sex (which might result in gendered experiences), or skin colour, appearance, and national origin (which might contribute to racialized experiences), the biology that underlies childhood is not a permanent trait. In its insistence that children are 'beings', there is a tendency in the new social studies of childhood to forget that children are *also* 'becomings' – childhood, empirically, is a transitional state. Second, all adults have experience of childhood, whereas membership of many social groups is more closed – for example, it is difficult to move between social classes, and even more difficult to move between racialized groups and genders. The tendency to discount adults' experiences childhood is widespread in the new social studies of childhood, leading to a situation where children's limited insight into the adult world is treated as being of no consequence for their rights and competences, but adults' insights into children's worlds are seen as being of little value. Moreover, that adults might base many of their views of childhood directly on remembered experiences of childhood (their own and others), rather than being dictated to by accounts of childhood offered by developmental psychology, seems to be rarely considered. Thus, while celebrating children's agency, adults' agentic capacities are downgraded.

Childhood cancer and families

The effort to 'liberate' the study of the child from the study of the family was perhaps necessary in order to distinguish children as objects of attention in their own right. We have two major reservations about the project to study children either independently of families or to study families solely from the perspective of the child. First, in approaching the social science study of childhood cancer, among the key reasons for being explicit about the location of the child within the family are the implications for the child's own experiences of childhood illness. As we shall show in this book, children's experiences are crucially shaped by their family context. Obtaining a diagnosis of childhood cancer, for example (Chapter 2), depends crucially on parents' actions and access to repertoires and resources that will avoid their child's symptoms being discounted. Similarly, children's experiences of communication (Chapter 6) and decision making (Chapter 7) are crucially affected by how their parents (or those with parental responsibility) behave.

Second, a key element of our criticism of the 'new' social studies of childhood is that, in its valorization of children, their perspectives, experiences and rights, it has neglected to consider how people who are not children experience childhood. Childhood, as a social state, affects not just children but adults. As Alanen (2001) points out, parents cannot exist structurally without children. We propose that parents' experiences of their children's childhoods must, therefore, be an object of social scientific attention. We further propose that analysis of experiences of childhood illness demonstrates that, although childhood is argued by many of those working within the new social studies to be a social state that oppresses children, it is in fact just as convincing to argue that the social state of childhood oppresses adults, particularly in the context of serious childhood illness.

The social constructionist movement within the sociology of childhood has been helpful in drawing attention to the socially constructed nature of childhood, and the implications of the 'dominant account' for children's experiences of childhood. We argue that parenthood is similarly socially constructed, with equally (if not more) powerful 'dominant accounts', and that there is an important need to explore the social construction of parenting in relation to serious childhood illness. Social constructions of parenthood are irrevocably tied to social constructions of childhood, including those that create childhood as a protectionist experience (Freeman 1997), and these create multiple, highly demanding, obligations for parents and other adults. Within contemporary Westernized cultures, the well-being of children is inextricably linked to the quality of parenting, and parents experience particular obligations to secure that well-being and face censure and possible legal redress if they fail. These include powerful pressures on mothers of children with serious illness and disability to conform to traditional ideologies of care in which they devote themselves selflessly to the welfare of their children (McKeever and Miller 2004). Although they are not themselves ill, parents experience many of the consequences of chronic illness, including biographical disruption, compromise in role function and deterioration in quality of life (Young et al. 2002).

Arguably, the kinds of oppression that children are supposed to experience – practices of regulation, control, surveillance, interference – apply equally, if not more intensely, to parents of severely ill children. However, thus far, most theorizing of childhood has been exclusively concerned with children's experiences of childhood, and explicitly sought to understand child–adult relations from the perspective of children. Adults' experiences of children's childhoods remain taken-for-granted or rendered uninteresting. For example, Brannen and O'Brien's (1996a) edited collection on children in families begins by emphasizing that there is no point in detaching children from their families, but many of the individual articles nonetheless were oriented towards the child in the family, rather than the child and the family. There is a chapter on conceptualizing parenting from the standpoint of children, but no chapter that conceptualizes childhood from the standpoint of parents. Alanen and Mayall's (2001) edited collection on child–adult relations similarly considers relations only from the perspective of children. Where parents have been studied, it has been via work on caring or in feminist accounts of motherhood, and although there are some excellent examples, parenthood and childhood have rarely been considered at the same time.

We argue that parents' and families' experiences are an important element of any attempt to produce a social science account of experiences of childhood cancer: to study 'doing childhood' without studying 'doing parenthood' is to risk producing a reified and partial account of experiences of childhood. We argue that an approach that neglects to locate the experience of childhood illness within the family is too limited, and insults the experiences of parents. We propose that what happens to children is not usually experienced by children alone, but has wider implications for the family in which they are being raised. Central to our analysis of the experience of childhood cancer is the need to understand the experiences of those socially and emotionally adjacent to children as well as children themselves, including siblings, grandparents, and so on, as well as parents.

We also recognize that there is the need to treat 'the family' as problematic at several levels. As units of social organization, the form and structure of families varies from society to society and within societies, and children may live, during the course of their childhood, in a number of different families. Moreover, families are not always a source of love and support for children, even seriously ill children, and the interests of those caring for children may not always coincide precisely with those of the children themselves. As Butler (1996) notes, the growing interest in the family as the site not only of nurture for its members but also of exploitation and abuse clearly argues for a differentiation of the interests of adults and children in thinking about families.

Psychological and developmental approaches to childhood and childhood cancer

As noted earlier, social science perspectives on childhood have long been dominated by the discipline of psychology: it has even been argued that childhood was constituted as a object of the scientific gaze primarily through this discipline (Scott et al. 1998). The dismissal of psychology as a legitimate means of studying childhood that is evident in much of the work in the new social studies of childhood seems to us misguided.

There are certainly a number of valid criticisms of traditional applications of psychology, particularly as it has been applied to the study of childhood cancer (as we outline below and elsewhere in the book), but to reject wholesale its potential contribution risks providing a partial, wholly social, account of childhood, and degrades the potential for social science research to contribute to measuring important outcomes of childhood cancer. Such measures are important, not least so that appropriate intervention can be provided during and after illness, but also in assessing the effects of intervention to treat childhood cancer – assisting, for example, in the context of clinical trials. We also argue that a science of development – one that can provide rigorous insight into the patterns of individual development within cognitive and emotional domains – is needed to complement socially based approaches.

Our concerns about dismissing psychology stem from several sources. Although critics of conventional developmental psychology correctly identify the influence of Piaget-like thinking on discourse, policies and practices in relation to childhood, it is worth noting that much of the critique of developmental psychology *as a discipline* is founded on something of a caricature. Those within the new social studies of childhood tend to see the discipline as directly and solely influenced by Piagetian theory and as endlessly recycling 'myths' about developmental stages, but developmental psychology is much more diverse than sociologists have generally given it credit for. Stage theory has been repeatedly challenged within developmental psychology, and Piaget is far from being regarded as the last word (Goswami 2002a). Some branches of developmental psychology have also been explicitly social in their orientation, and the work of Vygotsky (a contemporary of Piaget whose work only gained widespread influence in the 1970s) offered an early challenge to the notion that cognitive development is some kind of universal process, or that it can be studied apart from social and cultural processes. Like Piaget, Vygotsky's focus was on individual development, but unlike Piaget, at the heart of his work was a recognition that understanding child development requires an understanding of how mental processes originate and develop through social interactions and contexts, and of the mediating role played by socio-cultural tools, particularly language, in development (Rowe and Wertsch 2002).

Moreover, within psychology itself we have seen the growth of a social constructivist movement, which has advanced a wide-ranging critique of developmental psychology (for example, Burman 1994; Jenks 1996b). Within the social constructivist movement in psychology, there is much similarity with recent sociological conceptualizations of childhood in the basic underlying arguments (Morss 2002). The social constructivist approach proposes that development stems from the interactions of children with their social environment, and sees children as reflexive, critical and creative, actively monitoring, modifying and rejecting norms in the light of their experiences and knowledge.

Empirical work in psychology since the mid-1980s on children's understanding of emotional processes has demonstrated pre-school children's proficiency in understanding others' mental states (Wellman 2002) and has provided some support for certain elements of these theoretical approaches. Nonetheless, it is important to note that some of this work gives considerable importance to universal changes in children's abilities (Wellman 2002), and to crucial role played by age-related maturationally-based progression in children's abilities (Kagan 2003).

Finally, the assertion that it is Piagetian understandings of childhood that permeate practices and policies in relation to children is unproven. It is possible – even likely – that many practices, particularly parenting practices, are founded on direct observations of children and shared 'lay' knowledge of child-rearing, and perceptions of age-related abilities and other attributes may reflect stubborn realities rather than the effects of indoctrination with Piagetian thinking. These less formal forms of knowledge are likely to recognize that children's behaviours and competences vary by age, without necessarily being influenced by formal theory.

In this book we argue that the main 'problem' of psychology is that the social science study of childhood cancer has suffered by being dominated by this discipline. We argue that psychology is necessary, but we have several criticisms of its application so far to the study of the psychosocial sequelae of childhood cancer. Some of our criticisms relate to the execution of the research, with many examples of poor quality studies. Perhaps more importantly, our criticisms relate to how children and their families have come to be constructed within psychological studies of childhood cancer. Largely preoccupied with identifying and measuring psychopathology or psychoso-cial maladjustment in both children and parents, psychology has constituted childhood cancer as something that happens *to* people: children with cancer and their families are portrayed as the victims of psychologically, as well as physically, malign processes, prone to problems such as separation anxiety, social withdrawal, post-traumatic stress disorders, isolation, and dependency (Barakat et al. 2000). Within this discourse, people are then rendered as ob-jects, acted upon by external influences, rather than as subjects, capable of acting in the world and shaping responses to it. By focusing so relentlessly on issues of individual psychopathology, psychology has excluded the study of other important aspects of the experience of childhood cancer, and its pursuit of individual deficits has drawn attention from important mediators of the experience, such as social processes and access to resources.

Psychology has also tended to construct experiences of childhood cancer from an adult perspective that does no favours either to children or to their adult carers. There is a tradition within the psychology of childhood cancer of seeking the reports of parents as proxies for children. This practice has a doubly silencing effect, resulting in parents' voices being heard only as speaking on behalf of their children, and not on behalf of themselves, and children's voices being unheard. The unique moral and legal status of parents as guardians of their children's well-being and the complexity of their roles as caregivers, advocates and individuals in their own right is thus under-estimated, while there is also a failure to recognize children as 'beings' in their own right who have something to contribute to the characterization of their own experiences. It attributes the 'work' of caring for a child with cancer to adults (both parents and professional carers) and denies the important role that children have in producing their own health, for example in their en-during and strategic management of the arduous therapies involved in the treatment of childhood cancer.

Despite these criticisms, we argue that psychological approaches have an important role in studying experiences of childhood cancer. The problems thus far do not negate the validity of psychology as a disciplinary approach, and indeed a psychological approach is necessary to avoid the reification of experiences of childhood cancer as purely social and to provide a science of development.

The need for an multidisciplinary interpretive approach

Thus far we have summarized the new social studies of childhood and have offered a critique as it applies to the social science study of childhood cancer. We now argue that what is required is an interdisciplinary interpretive ap-proach. Such an approach to childhood cancer is needed for several reasons.

Interpretive approaches are consistent with one of our primary arguments, which is the need to attend directly to the experiences and views of those affected by childhood cancer, and to understand their experiences from their own perspectives. Research based on good quality qualitative research is needed to balance the current weight of quantitative psychological research, to give due attention to processes as well as outcomes and to provide the empirical foundations for theorizing.

What is a child? A note on terminology

It will be clear from the preceding discussion that the definition of 'a child' is not straightforward, but there is clearly a need for some form of heuristic device to allow us to discuss members of the social category of childhood. Alanen (2001) discusses a number of ways in which category membership might be understood, distinguishing between external definitions based on some attribute such as age, and approaches based on internal connections in children's relationships to the social world, which focus on the complex set of social processes through which some people are constructed as children while others are constructed as adults. While this latter proposal has considerable appeal, it is not operationally useful in a book such as this, especially in terms of readability. We will define (arbitrarily, we acknowledge), a child as someone aged under 18.

It is also worth noting in this context that some terms (such as 'adolescent') have drawn scorn from the new social studies of childhood (for example, Mayall 1998; Oakley 1994), for their implication that adolescents are people who are *becoming* adults. We also endorse the argument that treating 'adolescence' as a distinct stage of development with distinctive behaviours and attributes is flawed and problematic, and suggest that Fine's (2004) recent analysis of adolescence as a period when young people draw on 'repertoires' characteristic of both adulthood and childhood, while also creating cultural traditions that are specific to childhood, is especially helpful as a way of understanding this particular form of childhood. In various places in the book we do use the term 'adolescent' because that is what has been used in the primary text that we are discussing. We recognize that young people generally dislike this term and do not use it themselves (Mayall 2000), and we will preferentially use the term 'young people'. It will, for the sake of elegance of expression, be necessary to use 'children' as a generic term to include young people, on occasion.

Finally, issues of 'families' and 'parents' also require some kind of heuristic device in order not to complicate the text, even if the terms used conceal the conceptual complexity that underlies them. Children live in a variety of family arrangements, often split over more than one site, that change over time, and may recognize a range of people (biologically related to them or not) as having a parental relationship with them. Throughout much of this book we will not problematize these relationships, and will refer to 'families' as those people that children see as being members of their family, and 'parents' those people who see themselves or are seen by children as fulfilling a parental role.

The clinical background to childhood cancer

Though this book is primarily intended to be a social science text, it is important that discussions of experiences of childhood cancer are grounded in an understanding of the clinical issues. In this section we offer a brief review of the classification of childhood cancer, which forms the foundation for many of our later chapters.

Classification of childhood cancer

The types of malignant disease, or cancer, that appear in children are very different from those seen in adults, where carcinoma of the lung, breast, gut and skin predominate. The term 'carcinoma' refers to a malignant growth that microscopically resembles the mature tissue from which it has arisen. By contrast, childhood cancers commonly have the microscopic features of embryonal tissue (as normally seen in the fetus) and are given terms such as neuroblastoma (from nervous tissue) and nephroblastoma (from kidney). Classification of malignancies in children is, therefore, usually accomplished mainly on the basis of the histology (the cell types involved), rather than the primarily organ-based system used in adults.

The commonest childhood cancer is leukaemia (cancer of blood), responsible for a third of all cases, with most of these (approximately 80 per cent) being the acute lymphoblastic type. Of tumours arising from solid organs, brain tumours make up the largest group (24 per cent) with the remainder divided into those from bone (osteosarcoma), muscle (rhabdomyosarcoma), lymphatic system (lymphoma), kidney (Wilms' tumour), nervous tissue (neuroblastoma) and a group of less common tumours (Figure 1.1).

Leukaemia

Leukaemia is a malignant proliferation of precursor cells occurring in the bone marrow, resulting in replacement of the normal bone marrow cells with malignant cells that subsequently enter the blood stream. Acute lymphoblastic leukaemia (ALL) accounts for 80 per cent of leukaemias in children.

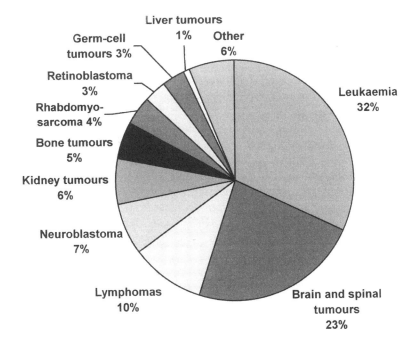

Figure 1.1 Prevalence of childhood cancers.

Most of the remainder are acute myeloid leukaemia (AML); chronic myeloid leukaemia is rare. Leukaemia as a group is the commonest malignancy of childhood and every year there are up to 2000 new cases of childhood ALL in the USA and approximately 350 in the UK. The peak age incidence for ALL is between 2 and 6 years with a slightly higher incidence in males.

ALL is always a widespread disease and requires intensive and prolonged chemotherapy treatment, which is systemic in nature (reaching all parts of the body). After an initial period of hospitalization, most of the subsequent treatment is administered as an outpatient and continues for between 2 to 3 years. Only a small percentage of patients require a bone marrow transplant and most can be cured with standard chemotherapy alone. The 5-year survival for ALL is now in the order of 80 per cent.

Brain tumours

Brain tumours are of special importance because they are the commonest solid tumour of childhood and because they cause extreme distress to the child and family during their often protracted natural history (Pinkerton and

Plowman 1997). Brain tumours form a spectrum from those that are slow growing and relatively benign to those that are highly malignant with a poor prognosis. Astrocytomas form 40 per cent of brain tumours and may either be low grade (slow-growing) or high grade. While localized astrocytomas in the cerebellum (the portion of the brain that coordinates movement of the voluntary muscles) usually have a good prognosis, those in other sites are often more difficult to treat, with a poorer prognosis. Medulloblastomas (20 per cent of brain tumours, and the second major group) are malignant tumours derived from primitive embryonal tissue and have a peak incidence in 5-year-olds. They require intensive multimodal treatment with surgery, radiotherapy and chemotherapy with a cure rate in the order of 60–70 per cent. Brain tumours present a major challenge for treatment in that the main problem is one of local control, and in an organ that is very sensitive to late treatment effects including brain damage with physical, emotional and learning disabilities.

Lymphoma

There are two main types of lymphoma: Hodgkin's disease (HD) and non-Hodgkin lymphoma (NHL). Together they comprise 10 per cent of childhood tumours and both arise from lymphoid tissue (part of the body's immune system). Both typically result in enlargement of lymph glands and may also spread to organs in the abdomen (liver and spleen) and to the bone marrow. NHL has a peak incidence between the ages of 7 to 10 years, while HD is commonest in adolescents. Lymphomas have proved amenable to chemotherapy and this is now the mainstay (rather than radiotherapy or surgery) and the prognosis is generally excellent.

Neuroblastoma

Neuroblastoma arises from neural crest tissue in the adrenal gland (in the abdomen) and from sympathetic nervous tissue in the chest and abdomen. Most children with neuroblastoma present under the age of 5. For reasons related to the biology of the disease, the prognosis in children under 1 year is often excellent, with some tumours undergoing spontaneous regression. However, after this age the situation is radically different and children often have widespread disease, are acutely ill and have an extremely poor prognosis with survival in the order of 20–30 per cent. Even with intensive treatment with prolonged hospitalization, the outlook for this cohort of children is poor.

Kidney tumours

Wilms' tumour (nephroblastoma) is the commonest kidney tumour. It arises from embryonal renal tissue and most cases present before the age of 5 years. The tumour responds well to chemotherapy and surgery is undertaken to remove the tumour mass together with the kidney from which it has arisen. The remaining kidney is usually healthy and most children do not develop renal failure. The prognosis is excellent with cure rates of more than 80 per cent, even for children who present with widespread disease and metastases in the lung. Treatment typically extends over a 3–6 month period.

Bone tumours

Sarcomas are cancers that develop in the supporting structures of the body (bone or soft tissue). Osteosarcoma is the most common malignant bone tumour and although occurring at any age, is most typically seen in the second decade, where it is linked with rapid bone growth. Ewing's sarcoma is commonest in the 10–15 year age group but is seen in younger children as well. Both bone cancers have higher prevalence in males. Most tumours occur in the limbs where persistent localized bone pain is a characteristic symptom, usually preceding the detection of a mass. However, an important sub-group includes those that occur in the spine and pelvis, where detection is much harder and there may be a long symptom interval before a diagnosis is made. These 'central' tumours are also harder to treat.

Both osteosarcoma and Ewing's sarcoma are difficult to treat, although the prognosis has improved in recent years and is of the order of 60–65 per cent depending on the site, the extent of spread and response to treatment. Initial evaluation must include careful assessment of the primary site to define the extent of the local disease, particularly with the likelihood of limb salvage surgery being contemplated. Treatment involves the use of combination chemotherapy given before surgery. There is increasing experience in avoiding amputation by using en bloc resection of the tumour with an endoprosthetic replacement. This allows preservation of the limb with an artificial prosthesis inserted, which often includes an artificial joint as well. Although this is cosmetically much more acceptable, it still places significant demands on children, involving rehabilitation, future surgery to lengthen the prosthesis as the child grows, and a range of late complications.

Rhabdomyosarcoma

Rhabdomyosarcoma originates from primary embryonal muscle or connective tissue. There are two peaks of incidence, the first and most important in children of 2–5 years of age, and the second during adolescence.

Rhabdomyosarcoma can occur virtually anywhere on the body. The commonest site is in the head and neck, causing, for example, proptosis (swelling of eye), nasal obstruction and blood-stained nasal discharge, polypoid mass in the ear, hoarseness of voice and difficulty breathing. The next most common site is the genito-urinary tract causing dysuria (pain or difficulty passing urine), bladder obstruction and a mass or discharge arising from the vagina. Initial assessment will focus on sites of tumour spread, as these greatly affect treatment and prognosis. For localized tumours that can be surgically removed, the prognosis is good (approximately 80 per cent with 5-year survival). For tumours with local spread a combination of surgery and intensive chemo-therapy is required, with a 5-year survival of approximately 65 per cent. If there is evidence of distant metastatic spread, the prognosis is poor despite attempts at aggressive therapy. Depending on the site of the tumour there is a risk of deformity resulting from the tumour and surgery.

Other childhood cancers

A range of other less common tumours exist in childhood requiring individualized and specialist treatment. Examples include retinoblastoma, a tumour of the eye occurring in young infants, germ-cell tumours (which develop from embryonal cells producing eggs or sperm), and liver tumours.

Epidemiology of childhood cancer

The reported incidence of childhood cancer varies worldwide (Parkin et al. 1998), probably depending on how the data are collected as well as reflecting genuine differences between populations. In the United Kingdom approximately 1500 new cases of childhood cancer are diagnosed each year. This equates to an incidence of 120–140 new cases per million children aged less than 15 years. Childhood cancer is approximately one fifth more common in boys.

There is some evidence of variation in cancers by social and ethnic group (Stiller 2004). The incidence of cancer is lower in black children, mainly because the incidence of ALL is about half that in white children (Parkin et al. 1998). There is some evidence of an elevated risk of childhood cancer in South-Asian populations in the UK (Cummins et al. 2001; Stiller et al. 1991). The incidence of ALL is in general correlated with levels of socioeconomic status with children from more affluent backgrounds more at risk (Stiller 2004), although the evidence on the relationship between social class and risk of childhood cancer is not conclusive in the UK (Dockerty et al. 2001), and for some tumours (for example, neuroblastoma and Hodgkin's disease), there is some evidence of increased risk for children in poorer socioeconomic conditions (Stiller 2004).

Some studies have demonstrated a small, but persistent increase in the incidence of childhood cancer (Cotterill et al. 2000; Dreifaldt et al. 2004). Some of the suggested increases in specific tumour groups, such as brain tumours, may be due to better reporting or may represent a true trend. Assessing incidence in adolescent cancers is challenging because they tend to be excluded from both child and adult cancer registries, but some evidence points to a substantial increases in the incidence of adolescents during the period 1973–95, due mainly to malignant germ-cell tumours and lymphoid neoplasms (Albritton and Bleyer 2003; Barr 2001).

Different tumour groups have specific age distributions. Acute leukaemia is commonest in children aged 2–3 years. A peak in early age is also seen in the typically 'embryonal' tumours such as neuroblastoma and Wilms' tumour. Adolescents have a distinctive pattern of cancers: tumours that occur commonly among younger children (retinoblastoma, neuroblastoma, Wilms' tumour, ependymoma, rhabdomyosarcoma, primitive neuroectodermal tumour (PNET) and hepatoblastoma) are hardly ever seen in adolescents and young adults (Gatta et al. 2003). Breast, colon and lung cancers (adult malignancies) rarely appear in adolescents (Bleyer 2002). Lymphomas are more common than leukaemias in the adolescent population, the reverse of the situation in those below 15 years of age (Gatta et al. 2003).

Causes of childhood cancer

Despite a huge body of research, the causes of childhood cancer remain largely unknown, There are only a few well-established environmental causes, including radiation. Only about 5 per cent of cases are thought to have an inherited component, though increasingly the association of many specific polymorphisms (gene variants) with childhood cancer is being identified (Stiller 2004). For those tumours with a peak incidence in early childhood and where the tumour resembles embryonal tissue, it is likely that causative factors exist before birth and possibly even before conception (Stiller et al. 2004). The exact nature of any factor remains speculative. Large population-based studies have shown no evidence for links with families living near nuclear power stations, or environmental radiation or from low exposure levels of electro-magnetic fields (Bithell et al. 1994). Infection is known to play a role in some cases of lymphoma. For children with leukaemia there are a number of theories providing a link to infection, including the suggestion that acute leukaemia may result from a lack of exposure to infection and a subsequent failure of the immune system (Stiller et al. 2004).

Prognosis

> I was a brand-new fellow in paediatric hematology-oncology, in July 1963, when I first cared for a child with acute leukaemia. By then, with chemotherapy we were able to induce temporary remissions in many patients, but none of them were cured ... A common approach among hematologists then was to give as little chemotherapy as possible, because the children 'will die anyway, so one shouldn't make them ill' ... Long-term survivors of childhood leukemia were so rare that I cannot recall a single conversation on the topic during my fellowship. Instead, the effects of death and dying on staff as well as families, became a major part of supportive care and an object of study.
>
> (Simone 2003: 627)

One of the most striking features of childhood cancer has been the dramatic improvement in prognosis for children diagnosed with cancer. In 2001 the death rate for childhood cancer in the UK was 300 children per year. Only 30 years previously, in 1969, there were 850 deaths. The improvements in survival are most graphically illustrated by childhood leukaemia. In the early 1960s virtually every child with leukaemia died.

The first attempts to introduce treatments were often criticized and regarded as unethical, but the cure rate for childhood leukaemia has climbed steadily and is now 80 per cent. A similar picture is true for lymphomas and Wilms' tumour. For bone tumours, brain tumours and neuroblastoma it has been more difficult to achieve similar results, but here too there have been improvements with survival for all these major groups being over 50 per cent.

Success in treating cancer in adolescents has not been as great as the success in treating cancer in younger children. The survival rates for many cancer diagnoses, including sarcoma and acute leukaemia, are lower in adolescents, with the degree of improvement smallest in the 15–19 age group (Bleyer 2002). The worst outcomes among the common cancers in 15- to 19-year-olds are in acute myelogenous leukaemia (AML), acute lymphoblastic leukaemia (ALL), and the sarcomas, particularly rhabdomyosarcoma, Ewing's sarcoma and osteosarcoma, where there are lower 5-year survival rates than that of the same malignancy in younger patients; thyroid carcinoma, melanoma and germ-cell tumours show a better prognosis (Albritton and Bleyer 2003).

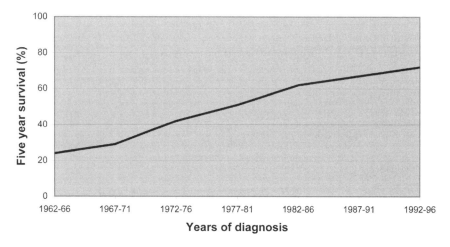

Figure 1.2 Trends in five-year survival rates for all childhood cancers from 1962 to 1996 (Great Britain).

Source: National Registry of Childhood Tumours

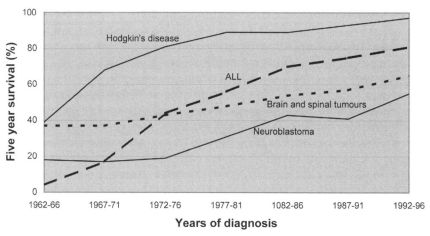

Figure 1.3 Trends in five-year survival rates for children diagnosed with selected tumours from 1962 to 1996 (Great Britain).

Source: National Registry of Childhood Tumours

Treatment

The outlook for an individual child depends on a range of factors, the most important of which are the type of tumour and the extent to which it has spread. Since the mid-1990s, the discovery of molecular events within the tumour cell have provided clues as to the cancer process and are now being incorporated in selecting prognostic groups and guiding treatment. Two concepts dominate the treatment of childhood cancer. The first is that treatment is multimodal, making use of different therapies and combinations of agents. The second is that treatment is delivered by a complex team of people. The structure of care delivery systems and the environment in which they are delivered are as important as the therapy itself and both have contributed to the improved prognosis.

Chemotherapy

Chemotherapy is now the backbone of most treatment protocols and makes use of cytotoxic drugs that are toxic to the cancer cells and interfere with proliferation and growth of the cancer. Similar drugs to those used in adult cancers are used, but in children appear to be more effective and offer a curative potential. Drugs are commonly used in combination and often used with other treatment modalities. The aim of chemotherapy is to kill all the cancer cells, and to achieve this the dose is often taken to the maximum tolerated level, with associated toxicity to the other parts of the body. Chapter 4, which outlines the late effects of treatment, includes tables with the names of the drugs and their expected toxicity.

A central venous line needs to be inserted to safely give the treatment. For example, a Hickman line (a thin plastic tube) may be inserted into a large vein under the collarbone, coming out of the skin on the chest wall. This stays in place for many months and allows children to have blood tests as well as providing a route for giving chemotherapy without having to subject children to frequent needle pricks. Chemotherapy inevitably means spending significant time in hospital and all drugs are associated with a long list of side effects. Treatment continues for a variable period depending on the type of tumour and may last anything from 6 months to 3 years. Some of the common complications include nausea and vomiting, hair loss, sore mouth, gut problems and bone-marrow suppression with anaemia, infections and bleeding. There are also many other organ specific complications.

Bone-marrow and stem-cell transplantation

Bone-marrow and stem-cell transplantation are used in situations where it is necessary to provide high-dose treatment that could be potentially lethal. The marrow or stem cells are used to reverse the life-threatening suppression of the bone marrow. These procedures carry a greater risk and are reserved for patients with high-risk disease where it is felt that standard chemotherapy will not be sufficient. Not only are there many short-term complications, but it has become clear since the mid-1990s that the long-term consequences, or 'late effects' of this treatment are also important (Chapter 4).

Radiotherapy

Radiotherapy makes use of ionizing radiation to cause cell damage or destruction and is targeted at the cancer. There has been a trend to reduce the use of radiotherapy in children as chemotherapy has become more effective. The one exception is brain tumours, where radiotherapy is still the mainstay of treatment, together with surgery. Radiotherapy requires daily hospital attendance for a period of 4–6 weeks. It has side effects that depend on the exact site affected but commonly include hair loss, sore mouth, sore skin and suppression of bone marrow. For radiotherapy to the brain additional consequences include impaired cognitive abilities and hormonal effects with reduced growth.

Surgery

Surgery has a number of roles and in the first instance is usually performed to obtain tissue for diagnosis. This may be followed at a later date by the removal of all or part of the tumour. Decisions on surgery involve a balance between extensive or mutilating surgery and what is required to provide the best opportunity for cure in combination with other treatments. Skilled perioperative care has helped reduce the surgical risks, but the long-term prognosis depends on many other factors.

Care delivery systems

We have noted earlier that we recognize diversity of family structures. It is also important to note diversity of access to treatment for childhood cancer, and to acknowledge that our analysis of experiences of childhood cancer is located within a westernized model of healthcare and societal organization. Within the UK treatment takes place in 22 designated childhood cancer treatment units. The centres are linked by an overarching organization, the United Kingdom Children's Cancer Study Group (UKCCSG) which brings together the health professionals involved, and provides protocols for treatment and guidelines for standards of care. Similar structures exist in the USA, Europe and other parts of the developed world. The advent of these specialized tertiary-care units and the fact that all children with cancer are now referred to them has been a major factor in the improved prognosis seen over the past 30 years. These centres may, however, be considerable distances from the children's homes. To support children closer to home there is a network of shared-care centres, which consist of local hospitals where a smaller designated team can provide a limited range of treatments.

Conclusions

Our main argument throughout this book is that the social science study of childhood cancer can benefit from multidisciplinary critical interpretive perspectives that can restore agency and reflexivity to children and to parents, and that are grounded in an understanding of the clinical issues. We have suggested that the study of childhood cancer has until recently been dominated by criteria of psychosocial adjustment and maladjustment. These do have important roles, but are too limited to provide full insight into experiences of childhood cancer. In concentrating largely on families who experience psychological problems arising from childhood cancer, the psycho-oncology tradition renders uninteresting other experiences, including the experiences of children and parents who do not experience lasting psychological difficulties. We propose that the experience of childhood cancer cannot be understood without considering key social processes, including how those who experience childhood cancer (children and their families) perceive and negotiate the disease, particularly in relation to issues such as identity, status and role.

This book will seek to move beyond approaches that endlessly catalogue families' difficulties. The new social studies of childhood provides a fresh and engaging perspective from which to theorize the experience of childhood cancer, but we must remain aware of some of the dangers of a straightforward application of current theory in the new social studies of childhood. The growth of the sociology of childhood should not involve a wholesale rejection of psychological approaches to the measurement of mental abilities, distress, quality of life, and other areas in which psychology has specialist expertise, nor should it involve a reification of childhood as distinct from parenthood. What is instead required is a holistic interdisciplinary approach that has as its core aim an understanding of how those affected by childhood cancer understand and organize their lives.

Note

1   It is interesting to note that traditionally sociology has been more unified than psychology in pursing this view of children as passive. For example, unlike his contemporaries the behaviourists, Piaget saw a crucial role for children's *intentional* actions on the environment in driving their learning (Smith 2002), though this point is generally not acknowledged by critics within the 'new' social studies of childhood.

2 Obtaining a diagnosis of childhood cancer

In this chapter we describe the ways in which childhood cancer typically presents and how it is diagnosed, and discuss research that has investigated families' experiences of obtaining a diagnosis of childhood cancer. The epidemiological, clinical and organizational context is essential in interpreting the social science literature. Childhood cancer is an uncommon disease: one child in every 550–600 can expect to develop cancer before the age of 15, and 150 new cases appear per million children per annum. The low incidence of childhood cancer poses significant challenges for its diagnosis, particularly in a primary-care-led system such as that which operates in the UK. A family doctor will, on average, see a child diagnosed with cancer once every 20 years (Feltbower et al. 2004). Many signs and symptoms of childhood cancer are non-specific, vague and have potentially innocent explanations, and the resulting low index of suspicion about the possibility of childhood cancer has significant implications for people's experiences of obtaining a diagnosis.

Symptoms of childhood cancer

The symptoms a child presents with depend on the type of tumour, the primary site and the biological behaviour of the tumour. Even for a single tumour type, there is a large range of presenting patterns. Some tumours are by nature indolent and slow growing, producing localizing signs over many months. More rapidly growing aggressive tumours may present with a short history of acute symptoms, and if there is metastatic disease there may be generalized features of weakness, lethargy, weight loss and pallor.

Leukaemia

Leukaemia commonly presents with a relatively short history of a few weeks or days. The primary problem in leukaemia is a malfunction of the bone marrow, and thereafter of the blood cells. This results in recurrent infections (because of a low white blood count), fatigue and pallor (because of anaemia) or bleeding (because of a low platelet count). Other symptoms may include irritability, bone pain, pallor, or bruising/pinpoint red spots on the skin. In addition children with leukaemia often have an enlargement of their liver or spleen and may have lymphadenopathy (swollen lymph glands). Many of the signs and symptoms of leukaemia commonly present in primary care in children without cancer, especially in children with infection. Lymphadenopathy poses particular problems because of the challenges of assessing its significance in children of different ages.

An assessment of a child presenting with symptoms suggestive of leukaemia would include a check of the liver/spleen and lymph nodes, and a blood test. A blood test in a child with leukaemia would reveal decreased red cells, low level of normal white blood cells, blasts (abnormal, immature white blood cells), and decreased platelets. A blood test with these findings is usually highly suggestive of the diagnosis and will trigger an urgent referral to hospital. A bone marrow test is required to confirm the diagnosis of leukaemia.

Brain tumours

The diagnosis of brain tumour is made using an MRI (magnetic resonance imaging) scan. The presenting features of a brain tumour depend on the anatomical location of the tumour. In childhood, 60 per cent of brain tumours are in the lower rear part of the brain (the cerebellum), directly above the brain stem. These tumours affect balance and eye movement, or commonly cause a blockage of the flow of cerebrospinal fluid with resulting raised intracranial pressure (ICP). Raised ICP causes headache and vomiting, especially early in the morning. While these are the classic features mentioned in all textbooks, many children present with a range of other less typical symptoms. These include ataxia (lack of coordination), squints, changes in personality and mood, out-of-character behaviour, developmental delay, weight loss and deterioration of school performance (Edgeworth et al. 1996). Again, many these symptoms may commonly present in primary care in children who do not have cancer. For children under the age of two years, an enlarging head circumference is seen with vomiting and unsteadiness (Gordon et al. 1995). For these very young children, this is often indicative of a late diagnosis, and the association of aggressive tumour biology and difficulties in treating young children make the prognosis particularly poor for this group.

Lymphoma (Hodgkin's disease and Non-Hodgkin's lymphoma)

Lymphomas cause swelling of lymph glands and symptoms will depend on local pressure from the tumour. Pain or swelling occurs at the site of the cancer, which in two-thirds of cases will be in the neck, chest or abdomen. Other symptoms include abdominal bloating, pain, weight loss, itchiness, night sweats, fever and change in bowel habits. In Hodgkin's disease the persistent swelling of a lymph gland in the neck is the most common scenario. Since this symptom frequently occurs with any infection of the throat or tonsils, there is often a period of observation. Non-Hodgkin's lymphoma is often extensive by the time the disease is diagnosed. Diagnostic imaging tests and a biopsy of tissue are normally required to make the diagnosis.

Bone tumours

Musculoskeletal malignancies pose particular challenges for diagnosis because musculoskeletal pain is a frequent symptom in children. Bone tumours typically present in adolescence, with leg (particularly the knee) or arm being the commonest sites. Persistent, localized bone pain is characteristic and is often present for some time before a lump is detected. If a lump is evident, the path to a diagnosis is clear. However, a significant number of primary tumours are in sites that are not obvious, such as the pelvis or spine. When this occurs, there is frequently a long preceding history with persistent pain and increasing disability for which no cause has been found, and often normal X-rays. If the tumour has been undiagnosed for a long time there may be symptoms of fever, loss of appetite, weight loss and severe night pain. A range of imaging equipment, including MRI, ultrasound, isotope and CT (computed axial tomography) scans may be used to make the diagnosis.

Abdominal tumours (Wilms' tumour, neuroblastoma, lymphoma, soft tissue sarcoma)

Wilms' tumour is the most common childhood kidney tumour, accounting for about 6 per cent of all paediatric cancers, and is one of the most successfully treated malignancies. The most common presentation is a symptomless abdominal mass – a typical story is that of a parent detecting a lump in the abdomen while bathing a young child. Identification of the mass by the family doctor usually leads to a quick referral to hospital. About a third of patients present with abdominal pain, anorexia, vomiting, malaise, or a combination of these symptoms (Kalapurakal et al. 2004), and these, along with other non-specific symptoms (which commonly appear in children without malignancies) including constipation, altered bowel and bladder habit, loss of appetite and behavioural changes, may be the presenting symptoms if the mass is not easily evident.

Some abdominal tumours may have metastatic features which are the first clue to an underlying problem. For example, neuroblastoma (adrenal tumour) may spread from the abdomen to the bone marrow and present with a low blood count. Diagnosis is usually made following abdominal ultrasonography and CT scan.

Other cancers

Tumours can affect almost any site in the body and there is an endless number of presentations. For example, rhabdomyosarcoma, a tumour of muscle origin, occurs in any site where muscle might be found, and consequently has diverse symptoms. Other cancers may have distinctive locations but vary in their signs and symptoms. The majority of retinoblastoma (cancer of the eye) cases, for instance, present with a white pupil reflex (leukocoria) rather than a normal black pupil or red reflex, but leukocoria is not always a symptom of cancer. Retinoblastoma can also present as a 'crossed' eye, as a red painful eye, as poor vision or inflammation of tissue surrounding the eye.

Presentation in primary care

Most childhood tumours present in primary care, but even if a family doctor were to see more than the national average, it is unlikely that he or she would see two children with the same malignancy in the course of his or her career. Since much clinical work is dependent on pattern recognition in relation to symptoms and signs, it is impossible for family doctors to make a diagnosis based on specific experience. However, family doctors have experience of normal presentations and the variations caused by common, but more minor, illnesses; the challenge is to recognize when the features no longer fit a simple diagnosis.

It will be evident from the discussion thus far that many symptoms of childhood cancer are very similar to those of much less sinister diseases. However, there is little good quality evidence to show the extent to which it is possible easily to distinguish between children with cancer and children with the same symptoms who do not have cancer. Cabral and Tucker (1999) reported a retrospective review of the records of 29 children who had been diagnosed with cancer following referral to two paediatric rheumatology centres. Children in this study showed features typical of many rheumatic disorders, including musculoskeletal pains, fever, fatigue, weight loss, hepatomegaly and arthritis. However 19 children (66 per cent), had one or more investigations with abnormal results suggestive of malignancy and clinical features 'atypical' of most rheumatic disease which were not recognized as abnormal in 11 patients (40 per cent), suggesting defects in the recognition of childhood cancer. Other studies have looked at the extent to which musculoskeletal pain, a non-specific symptom that is the presenting symptom of childhood cancers (for example, bone tumours, muscle sarcoma, leukaemia), is predictive of cancer. A review of 1254 patients attending a paediatric rheumatology unit in Italy over a 10-year period found an underlying neoplasia in 10 cases, and recommended that disproportionate levels of pain or atypical patterns of 'arthritis' should alert doctors to a possible tumour diagnosis (Trapani et al. 2000). However a review of 317 children presenting in a primary-care setting with very similar symptoms found no cases of malignancy (De Inocencio 2004).

The problems of trying to distinguish symptoms of cancer from symptoms due to other causes are well illustrated by the example of headache. Headache is an important symptom of brain tumours and at least 60 per cent of children with a brain tumour will have reported headaches. In a retrospective study of 74 children with a primary brain tumour presenting to a neurosurgical unit, the most common symptoms were vomiting (65 per cent) and headache (64 per cent) (Edgeworth et al. 1996). The problem with headache is that it is a non-specific symptom with high frequency of presentation, and in only a tiny fraction of these presentations is childhood cancer the underlying cause (Meloff 1982). Some 15–20 per cent of school-age children experience headache (Sillanpaa et al. 1991; Virtanen et al. 2002). If children are asked directly, up to 60 per cent will report having headaches (Sweeting and West 1998). It is extremely difficult to distinguish brain tumour headaches from benign headaches. Classically brain tumour headaches are reported to occur with vomiting and to be present upon waking in the morning. However, Edgeworth et al. (1996) found that 34 per cent of tumour headaches were not associated with vomiting and only 28 per cent occurred in the 'early morning'. In this study, migraine was initially diagnosed in 24 per cent of the children and a psychological aetiology in 15 per cent. A Swiss study (Dobrovoljac et al. 2002) based on 252 children diagnosed with brain tumours reported that the median symptomatic interval before diagnosis was 60 days (range 0–3010 days) with a parental 'delay' of 14 days (range 0–2310 days) and a doctor 'delay' of 30 days (range 0–3010 days). Only a third of these tumours were diagnosed within a month of the onset of symptoms.

Several attempts have been made to provide guidelines for family or hospital doctors to select those children who require further assessment (Annequin et al. 2000; Miles 2000). As part of a national initiative to improve the diagnosis of all cancers in adults and children the UK, government has introduced a policy for all patients with suspected cancer to be seen at a referral hospital within a 2-week period, and guidelines to help general practitioners recognize tumours at an earlier stage (Department of Health 2000). It is uncertain, as yet, whether this has made any difference to the diagnosis of cancer in children.

Making the diagnosis

Once a child has been referred to a specialist centre with a suspected diagnosis a series of events take place to determine the precise diagnosis, including a range of investigations and tests (see Box 2.1). Because of the huge implications of the illness, medical staff aim to be absolutely certain of the labels they propose to attach and have as much information available as possible.

Box 2.1 Investigations used in determining a diagnosis of childhood cancer

Blood tests, including a full blood test (FBC) is used to analyse the three major types of cells in the blood – red blood cells, white blood cells, and platelets.

Biopsy involves the removal and examination of tissue, cells, or fluid.

MRI (magnetic resonance imaging) uses radio waves and a strong magnetic field to provide detailed images of organs and tissues and can be used to produce images of some structures that may not be visible using other techniques.

Bone scan involves injection of radioactive material which accumulates in areas of cancer or infection in the body, which can then be detected using a special camera.

Ultrasound scans use high frequency sound waves to produce dynamic images of organs, tissues, or blood flow within the body.

Radiographs (x-rays) produce images by passing controlled doses of radiation through the body.

CT (computed tomography) scans are a form of x-ray imaging procedure and produce images of organs, tissues, or blood vessels.

Lumbar puncture involves removal of a small amount of the fluid that surrounds the spinal cord and brain (the cerebrospinal fluid).

Bone marrow aspirate involves the removal of bone marrow fluid through a needle inserted into the bone. A bone marrow biopsy is often done at the same time.

As well as diagnosis, the cancer or tumour will be *staged* to determine how advanced the malignancy is. Cancers are assigned a stage of I, II, III or IV based on the size of the cancer and how far from the original site the tumour has spread. Staging systems vary, but essentially involve determination of whether the tumour has remained local, or has spread to nearby body organs or glands or has spread to distant parts of the body. Cancer which has spread to a distant site is termed metastatic disease.

Leukaemia, however, is not usually staged because it already involves all the bone marrow in the body and has often spread to other organs. Testing for leukaemia involves evaluating the prognosis of the disease and determining which treatments will produce the best response. Prognosis will depend on sex, age, white blood cell count, genetics, the extent to which the central nervous system is involved, the immunology of the leukaemia cells, and early response to therapy. Further tests on tissue samples look at molecular markers that can help to guide treatment or indicate the prognosis. As this information is gained the medical team will start to think about treatment and a further set of investigations is required to evaluate the patient's general condition and function of key organs such as liver, heart and lung, before any treatment can be started.

Investigations to characterize the cancer and conduct staging can take a number of days and in many cases a few weeks to complete because of the nature of the tests involved. The consequence of this series of events is that the families often have a significant period from the time they are admitted to a specialist unit to the time treatment can be finally started. In some emergency situations treatment can be started in a relatively short time, but for most families there is ongoing uncertainty, anxiety and discussions with staff as more information becomes available.

Delay in diagnosis

The duration from the onset of symptoms to the diagnosis of cancer is known as the lag time. Studies examining lag time in childhood cancer have been reported from the UK, USA and Europe (Pollock et al. 1991; Saha et al. 1993; Thulesius et al. 2000), and have produced variable estimates. What they do demonstrate is that type of cancer and the ease with which it can be detected powerfully influences the lag time. Children whose presenting symptoms are pain, discomfort, or behavioural alterations, and with tumours that are not detectable on plain X-rays, are particularly prone to delay in diagnosis. Lag time appears to be shortest for leukaemia and Wilms' tumours, and longer for solid tumours (especially brain tumours). A recent study in Liverpool, UK (Ibrahim 2004) reported that in children with a brain tumour whose presenting symptom was seizure, there was a delay in diagnosis from two weeks to two years with a mean of six months. Bone tumours were reported by Pollock et al. (1991) to have a lag time of 11.5 to 20.8 weeks. A recent Israeli study of childhood malignancies (excluding leukaemia) (Haimi et al. 2004) reported a mean overall lag time of 15.75 weeks (range 0–208 weeks), with a mean 'parent delay' of 4.42 weeks (range 0–130 weeks) and a mean 'doctor delay' of 11.17 weeks (range 0–206 weeks). The mean lag time and doctor delay in disseminated disease were longer than in localized disease. In this study, the longest lag times occurred in relation to brain tumours and bone tumours, and the shortest in children with Wilms' tumour.

Age is a significant factor in delays in diagnosis, with older children presenting later. There are also regional variations, suggesting that the structure of the health system is an important determinant (Saha et al. 1993). The evidence on the impact of lag time on outcome is currently ambiguous. Some studies indicate no direct link in the majority of childhood cancers between the lag time and survival (Halperin et al. 2001; Saha et al. 1993), while others (Hamre et al. 2000) suggest that early detection of childhood cancer may be associated with reduced mortality. There are likely to be important sub-group differences.

Experiences of obtaining a diagnosis of childhood cancer

There is a small but important literature reporting on people's experiences of obtaining a diagnosis of childhood cancer, mostly using interview-based techniques. Most studies have reported parents' accounts: very little of the literature reports accounts from children. This could be attributed to a failure to seek the accounts of children or understand their perspectives. However, it is more likely to be due to a more complex set of methodological issues. First, accounts of obtaining a diagnosis must be gathered retrospectively, as it would be practically impossible to identify children who were going to be diagnosed with cancer in advance. Methods such as ethnography are, therefore, not possible. Second, there are sensitivities and possible ethical problems in exploring children's and young people's experiences of the events leading up to diagnosis. Third, while methods for gathering and analysing narratives from adults is well recognized, it is unclear as yet whether children's narratives are of the same form and lend themselves to the same types of approach.

Our own experiences illustrate the difficulties. As part of an interview-based study of children's, young people's and parents' experiences of childhood cancer we included a prompt to ask participants to tell us about the cancer from the beginning. While parents offered extremely detailed and lengthy accounts of the period leading up to diagnosis (Dixon-Woods et al. 2001), children did not discuss the period at all or spoke of it only very briefly, and young people tended, when asked about this issue, also to be brief and to give prominence to their parents' roles in obtaining the diagnosis. We did not feel comfortable about 'digging' any further for data on this issue. So little data were available as a result that it proved impossible to conduct an analysis, and we focused solely on reporting parents' accounts instead. It is likely that similar problems will affect other studies of this type. However, parents' accounts in our study and in others reported in the literature do offer significant insights into children's experiences as well as their own, suggesting that sometimes people other than children themselves are appropriate and important in providing data about children.

The literature on parents suggests that the pre-diagnosis period is one of enormous significance for them. For families who perceive a delay in diagnosis, this period not only heralds their biographical transition from 'normal' family to family in crisis, but is also a traumatic and anguishing period that persists in their narratives often many years after the events. Taken together, studies of obtaining a diagnosis of childhood cancer suggest that parents' narratives (particularly where there is a delay) have the following typical features:

- The narratives are organized around a biography or career of the child's illness, are highly detailed and begin at the beginning.
- Parents' own intuitive insight based on their detailed, intimate and unique experiental knowledge of their child 'tells' them something is seriously wrong.
- Parents are initially deferential in their interactions with doctors and accept their early actions and judgements.
- Health professionals are located in a discrete, separate, distinct world where they are powerful and placed in a position where they can adjudicate on the credibility of parents' accounts and the authenticity of the symptoms being presented as warranting investigation.
- In this other world, parents' knowledge is of low status and is discounted, often repeatedly. Biological abnormalities are prioritized by doctors over this intuitive, experiental knowledge.
- Temporalizing strategies are often used by doctors, who instantly reach for more common or more innocent explanations for the child's symptoms.
- Doctors may also use explanations that are potentially discrediting: for example, a psychiatric, behavioural or psychological problem in the child, or neurotic qualities in the parents, and these result in further delays.
- When investigations are initiated, they are often the wrong ones, or are handled or interpreted incompetently.
- As their child's condition worsens, parents may take on an advocacy role, using a range of strategies to try to secure investigations of their child, and subverting 'normal' routes.

It is evident that there is considerable variability in decisions on when to seek help. Eiser's study (Eiser et al. 1994) of 28 mothers and 23 fathers identified a mean of 17 weeks (range 1 week to 15 months) between parents first realizing that their child was ill and going to the doctor, until the diagnosis was made. There is some evidence that parents who delay in consulting experience guilt and remorse (Comaroff and Maguire 1981), but consulting behaviour is likely to depend on the way in which the disease presents. As we have described earlier, the onset of many childhood cancers is highly insidious and the symptoms are non-specific, meaning that they are likely to be attributed, at least initially, to trivial illness or other 'innocent' explanations. A number of studies (Dixon-Woods et al. 2001; Holm et al. 2003) have shown that families distinguish between medical symptoms, including earache, vomiting, sore throats, pain, loss of coordination, fits and difficulty with urination, and more intuitive, experientially-based insights into their own child's 'normal' behaviour and well-being, including changes from being a normal happy child, becoming highly emotional, becoming very quiet and losing 'boisterousness', and becoming very tired. In providing these accounts parents provide vivid insights into the experiences of their children in the period leading up to diagnosis, including the pain, disability, and withdrawal from social life that children sometimes endure. As we have already discussed, without accounts from children themselves, these experiences would remain hidden.

In terms of initiating consultations, Dixon-Woods et al. (2001) found that parents distinguished between the significance they assigned to different symptoms. The first and most common type of symptoms were those for which 'innocent' explanations – viral infection, muscle strain, wanting to get out of school, constipation, or developmental stage – were available. Parents tended to feel that symptoms such as tiredness, crankiness, and viral-type infections could be managed at home for a few weeks, but if symptoms persisted they should be investigated thoroughly and quickly. The second group of signs and symptoms consisted of unusual or frightening events, including fits, fainting, loss of coordination or balance, or blood in urine, which parents judged abnormal. These symptoms sometimes began to appear after innocent-type symptoms had been present for some time, and made parents feel more strongly that investigation was urgently required.

These accounts suggest that parents actively monitor and manage symptoms and initiate help-seeking when they deem that 'innocent' explanations for their child's condition can no longer be sustained. Importantly, the evidence suggests that it is parents, for the most part, who initiate consultations and manage much of the negotiations that follow, rather than children. This work also shows that the role of parents and the extent to which they can directly observe variations from normal vary according to the age and maturity of the child. For younger children, parents are very likely to be the first to notice something amiss – for example, they may feel an abdominal mass while bathing the child. Parents may, however, have few opportunities to see older children or young people without their clothes or to engage in close physical contact, and may have to wait to be told about symptoms. The reluctance of young people to consult may help to explain the finding that they are often diagnosed later (Saha et al. 1993).

> Yes, it was November when she first came to me and showed me her foot, and I felt awful because normally when your children are small you inspect them regularly, but once they get to be a teenager you're not allowed in the bathroom when they're in there, so I hadn't noticed there was anything wrong...
>
> (Mother of child C18 (solid tumour), quoted in
> Dixon-Woods et al. 2001: 671)

Parents in our study (Dixon-Woods et al. 2001) described the initiation of consultations for younger children as unproblematic. However, negotiations with older children were sometimes necessary in order to persuade them to visit a family doctor.

> ... she's not like an active girl like running about because inside she'd got pain but she didn't tell me she had this pain. And I am asking 'are you sure you're all right?' She says 'yeah'. I said 'are you sure you don't want to go to the doctor's ...?' She says 'no mum you really worry too much, I'll be all right.'
>
> (Mother of child C8 (leukaemia), quoted in
> Dixon-Woods et al. 2001: 672)

After consultations are initiated, accounts from parents generally fall into two categories: those that involve disputes with doctors and those that do not. Prompt referral and investigation is most likely to happen when a simple blood test can point to evidence of malignancy, or when there is a very evident lump or other unusual and highly suggestive symptom, but other presentations may be more prone to delay. In studies by Dixon-Woods et al. (2001) and Arksey and Sloper (1999), over half of families felt that there had been some avoidable delay in getting a diagnosis. Many report that parents made repeated visits to doctors in an increasingly desperate attempt to obtain a diagnosis (Dixon-Woods et al. 2001; Edgeworth et al. 1996; Eiser et al. 1994).

When disputes develop over the significance of children's symptoms, parents increasingly reject 'common-sense' diagnoses on the basis of the unusual nature of the symptoms and their intimate knowledge of their child. A common finding in studies of delays is that parents feel that the authenticity and credibility, not only of their child's symptoms, but also of themselves, are challenged by doctors. Dixon-Woods (2001) and Holm et al. (2003) describe how parents function as advocates in seeking a diagnosis for their child, and how, in some cases, they faced being discredited by professionals in their attempts to secure investigations. Their experiential knowledge of their child's normal condition is discounted as a resource in negotiating with healthcare staff; they report not being taken seriously and being told that they are neurotic. Parents see themselves as being excluded from a medical world in which biological signs and symptoms are the sole signals of illness, and their experience is relevant only in so far as it provides data about the abnormality (Armstrong 2003). Many parents report feeling overpowered in the doctor–patient relationship and unable to insist on having referrals or tests. Parents experience the spoiling of their identity as credible, rational people, and their apparent failure to act as effective advocates on behalf of their children as an acute and highly distressing form of suffering. Interestingly, parents' accounts provide insight into how older children and young people can also experience this form of discrediting:

> We went back to our family doctor several times because this didn't get any better, and didn't get any better. And then we saw different doctors in the group. We saw one doctor that was very short with [daughter's name] and shamed her, and that was very hard. I still, to this day, I still am really trying to forgive this doctor for being so shaming of our daughter.
>
> (Mother of 16-year-old complaining of sore shoulders, quoted in Holm et al. 2003: 306)

Parental persistence and advocacy – returning repeatedly, insistence, and using a range of subversive strategies, including use of private medicine and seeing multiple doctors – are reported as key to eventually ensuring that the correct investigations are undertaken (Dixon-Woods et al. 2001; Holm et al. 2003; Levi et al. 2000). In some cases, the diagnosis is made only when a medical crisis, such as kidney failure, occurs (Dixon-Woods et al. 2001).

In studies of apparent delays in diagnosis of childhood cancer, the view that it could and should have been detected earlier appears to be a universal one: for example, a study of Taiwanese parents (Yeh 2003) reported that anger at 'late' diagnosis was frequent among parents. Whatever the reality about the effects of lag time on survival, social science research indicates that parents absorb societal discourses about the need for early detection of cancers, and this means that they find it difficult to accept that any delay in diagnosis is of little consequence to their child's survival (Arksey and Sloper 1999). These effects may be especially pronounced if the cancer is advanced at the time of diagnosis, or if the child subsequently dies.

It might be thought likely that these poor experiences during the pre-diagnosis period would permanently damage families' trust and confidence in the medical profession, but the evidence suggests otherwise. Most parents appear to confine the blame to the individuals involved in this period (Dixon-Woods et al. 2001). It is probable that, once the diagnosis has been made, it is very necessary for families to believe in the medical profession as a source of salvation for their child, and parents then become focused on their relationships with staff involved in the care of their child rather than those who were involved before then. There is no doubt, however, that parents remain angry and distressed about what happened during this crucially important beginning of their biography as parents of a child with cancer.

To what extent delays in diagnosis are avoidable is unclear, given, as we have already described, the rarity of childhood cancer and the difficulties of distinguishing many of the symptoms from those of much less sinister childhood illnesses. A family doctor may see 20 children a week who are irritable and tired, but only one child over the course of his or her entire career with these symptoms that turn out to be those of leukaemia. Sometimes, too, parents insist that there is something wrong when in fact there is not, and family doctors are (understandably) reluctant to commit resources and to put children through often painful and distressing procedures simply to prove that the diagnosis is not cancer. One way of improving matters might be to ensure that referral practices and pathways are well coordinated and based on best available evidence. No standard guidance on when children should be referred for a brain scan currently exists, for example, even though brain tumours are particularly prone to lengthy delays in diagnosis in children. What appears to be more important, however, and what is evident in studies of parents' accounts, is the ways in which forms of professional–patient relationships tend to disadvantage people who are convinced, for reasons they may not be able to articulate very clearly, that there is something wrong with their child. These accounts need to be analysed on two levels: first, to explore the structure and status of the accounts, and second, how to explain why families appear to find professional–patient interactions so difficult to negotiate.

The importance of attending to the narrative properties of parents' accounts is evident from Baruch's (1981) work. Baruch argues that 'atrocity stories' are central to the ways in which people describe their encounters with health professions. Baruch notes a number of characteristics of these stories: they refer to events that have taken place early in the child's medical career, and they refer to conflict and disagreement, with health professionals casting doubt on the competence and rationality of parents. Schutz's (1962, 1964, 1966) analysis of common sense, in which common sense is understood as a system of typifications involving typical issues, typical solutions and typical actors, is invoked to explain how parents construct their accounts. There is considerable evidence of such typifications being used in parents' accounts to show how the delay in diagnosing their child's cancer represents a failure by health professionals. In most accounts, parents show how their initial interactions with health professionals rely on what Schutz describes as standardized recipes for action (for example, assuming initially that their child's symptoms are those of minor illness), but they are later forced to discard their familiar typifications and move to new, altogether more challenging and frightening ways of proceeding, which may themselves draw on other typi-fications.

One argument is that these accounts should be treated, on one level, as evidence of parents' attempts to demonstrate their moral character as com-petent, adequate parents (Baruch 1981). Baruch's arguments resonate with those of Goffman (1959), who describes how people's accounts may involve forms of impression management in order to protect their self-image or sta-tus, and later writers including Coffey and Atkinson (1996), who encourage researchers to reveal the devices used in constructing accounts. It is certainly true that in presenting narrative accounts, families may render events as much more orderly than they appeared at the time, and attach different meanings to events, perhaps, for example, seeing some symptoms as more significant than they seemed when they first presented. They may also talk about their experiences in different and apparently contradictory ways (West 1990). However, while attending to the ways in which parents produce ac-counts may be one way in which the accounts can be analysed, accounts should not be read solely as demonstrations of adequate parenthood. They also, and more importantly, offer significant insights into the experiences of people seeking to obtain a diagnosis of childhood cancer, and analysis of medical records suggests that many of the accounts they give are largely accurate as medical histories (Dixon-Woods et al. 2001).

Sociological theory about the doctor–patient relationship can help to explain why it is so difficult for parents to succeed in getting doctors to take symptoms seriously and problems in parents' intimate, experientially based knowledge of their child being discounted. Goffman (1967), Strong (1983) and Manning (1992) proposed that tacit rules of conduct simultaneously regulate and constitute the structure of social interaction. These rules are of two types: substantive (formal rules expressed in law or codes of conduct), and ceremonial (less formal rules that can be seen as 'rules of etiquette'). These latter rules govern polite, face-to-face interaction and function to maintain social order. Rules of conduct may express differential power dis-tribution – for example allowing one person authority over another. Strong (1979) argued that the 'ceremonial order' of doctor–patient relationships masks power differentials between doctor and patient through the imperative to maintain an apparently harmonious enounter. The ceremonial order makes it difficult for patients to mount direct criticism of doctors or to be seen to 'force' doctors to take a particular action. For parents who suspect there is something seriously wrong with their child, the ceremonial order may act as an extremely powerful brake on their ability to negotiate access to in-vestigations: they risk being seen as behaving illegitimately if they attempt to take control, and their main resource (their own knowledge of their child) is of low status. Their attempts at advocacy involve breaking ceremonial rules and are a costly and risky strategy.

Disclosure of diagnosis

As we have described earlier, it may take some time, because of the inherently lengthy nature of the tests, to establish a definitive diagnosis of cancer even when it has been strongly suspected and the investigations initiated. This 'waiting and not knowing' period has been described as extremely distressing for families (Clarke-Steffen 1993b). Even though families may have had a growing sense of something seriously amiss in the days, weeks, or months before diagnosis, its confirmation is often deeply shocking. Like the period leading up to diagnosis, parents often recall the disclosure in vivid detail and may remain preoccupied with it for many years (Woolley et al. 1989), though a study of parents of children with a range of conditions associated with physical disability indicated that satisfaction with disclosure was not a major determinant of long-term satisfaction with life or adaptation (Sloper and Turner 1993).

It is clear that disclosing a diagnosis of a serious, potentially fatal, illness to a child's parents is extremely difficult for all parties. In a study involving interviews with parents of 23 children with cancer, Eden et al. (1994) reported that in all cases the parents were the first members of the family to be informed of the diagnosis. All parents reported devastation, shock, numbness and anger. Eleven families felt they had not taken in what had initially been said. Nine families said they wished to have other people involved, but fourteen were adamant that they alone should be advised of the diagnosis, to give them time to come to terms with it before discussing with other members of the family. Eiser et al. (1994) reported that parents may feel unable to ask questions at the initial interview, even when encouraged to do so. The management of the disclosure for adolescents may be experienced as particularly problematic. Kelly et al. (2004) describe how adolescents react to the diagnosis with feelings of shock, intensified as many are just beginning to establish some degree of independence, as well as with an acute sense of uncertainty.

The disclosure of the diagnosis is clearly a key transitional point in the biography of the child's illness and the family. Clarke-Steffen (1993a), in a longitudinal study of seven families including children, parents and siblings, describes the diagnosis as a fracturing of reality, followed by a need to reconstruct reality in the light of chronic uncertainty. Dixon-Woods et al. (2001) found that parents' reactions to diagnosis of cancer were affected by their experiences of obtaining the diagnosis. Some parents who had had to struggle to get their child investigated felt vindicated or relieved, and that cancer was at least an identifiable diagnosis for which something could be done. At the other extreme, parents whose child was diagnosed within hours or days were shocked and stunned, and described feelings of numbness and disbelief. Parents who had had disputes commented at length on their role in getting the diagnosis, and some felt guilty and self-reproachful because they had not been more effective advocates for their child:

> If there was anything wrong with any of my children slightly that way I'd take action a lot quicker. I wouldn't let it go on as long as I did. I mean I wished I'd pushed the doctor at the GP's a bit more at the time.
>
> (Mother of child C9 (solid tumour), quoted in Dixon-Woods et al. 2001: 673)

Similar findings were also reported by Eden et al. (1994), who found that three families expressed guilt that they had not looked after their child properly, while five mothers expressed relief as they finally felt that they were being taken seriously by the medical profession.

Conclusions

Experiences of obtaining a diagnosis have mostly been studied through the retrospective accounts offered by parents. Their accounts offer witness not only to their own experiences, but also to those of their children, who to date have not generally been reported to offer their own detailed accounts of the pre-diagnosis period. To interpret parents' accounts, we draw attention to the very specific nature of illness narratives. Parents' accounts should be treated as narratives with functions other than to provide a strictly accurate and objective history. While to some extent these narratives need to be analysed as demonstrations of adequate parenthood (for example, it is notable that failures to listen to children or take their symptoms seriously are rarely reported) for the most part they can be seen to offer important insights into experiences of the period leading up to diagnosis. These accounts are constructed, but they are not fabricated, a point underscored by the consistency we noted between parents' accounts and notes in medical records (Dixon-Woods et al, 2001).

The diverse and unpredictable ways in which childhood cancer can present mean that early diagnosis is difficult. The rarity of childhood cancer compounds the situation. Faced with common symptoms that have a more probable explanation, doctors are unlikely to order invasive or expensive investigations. These features of the presentation of childhood cancer can conspire to cause forms of suffering for the children and their families. Doctors, therefore, risk appearing incompetent in accounts of obtaining a diagnosis of childhood cancer, even when they are acting reasonably. What does appear to be avoidable, however, is the form of suffering involved when parents perceive that their main claim to status in the consultation – their intimate knowledge of their child – is discredited. Discrediting this claim results in parents feeling that they lack a warrant for their consulting behaviour, and pushes them into desperation as the tension between their insight into their child's condition and the medical response to it appear increasingly out of alignment. An analysis of the accounts of professionals involved in protracted or delayed diagnoses is strikingly absent and would most likely be very informative.

3   Having childhood cancer

Comaroff and Maguire (1981) note that a diagnosis of childhood leukaemia taxes a family's sense of sharing in a common universe or experience. Families move through the transitional state of awaiting a diagnosis, described in Chapter 2, to one in which their taken-for-granted world is permanently altered. How children and their families experience childhood cancer is a key empirical and theoretical question. In this chapter we focus on children's and young people's experiences; those of families are discussed in Chapter 5, though, of course, neither the two sets of literatures nor the two sets of experiences are as distinct as such an organization of material might imply.

We begin by sketching in briefly the clinical background to treatment, which is necessary as a context for our subsequent discussion of social science approaches to exploring experiences of childhood cancer. To date, much of the research on people's experiences has been conducted within fairly rigid disciplinary boundaries, and within those boundaries has tended to tackle particular themes. Psychological approaches to the assessment of psychological well-being have dominated the study of childhood cancer, but there is an important and growing body of work using interpretive perspectives and methodologies, much of it conducted within a nursing paradigm. We will offer a critique of this work with particular reference to the relevance of theory from the sociology of chronic (adult) illness.

Treating childhood cancer

Understanding experiences of childhood cancer requires that we understand the clinical context of its management. Much of the improved survival of children with cancer can be attributed to increasingly effective treatment, but this is intensive and complex, and very often aggressive and arduous. The drive to improve the prognosis has resulted in a willingness to accept significant morbidity and toxicity that would be almost unthinkable in other medical contexts. Children are often acutely ill, spending prolonged periods in hospital, and are dependent on expert nursing care with input from specialized staff including physiotherapists, pharmacists, dieticians, play therapists, psychologists and a host of medical sub-specialists. Very many children will be treated as part of a clinical trial, and their treatment will be conducted according to a highly specified protocol, which will indicate precisely what treatments should be given and when. There are, generally speaking, two major phases of treatment: remission induction and remission maintenance. The first aims at reaching a stage where cancer cells are no longer detectable in the body; the second at maintaining this state, a process that may go on for months or even years.

Typical procedures in the treatment of childhood cancer

The precise combination of treatments that a child with cancer will undergo depends on the type of tumour, its location, its stage, and how well it responds to therapy. The mainstays of treatment in childhood cancer include chemotherapy, radiation therapy, surgery, and bone marrow and peripheral stem-cell treatment, but other treatments are also used, and a wide range of interventions, from blood transfusions to insertion of central venous lines, are required to support the main therapies.

Chemotherapy

Chemotherapy uses powerful drugs that interfere with the capacity of cancer cells to divide and multiply themselves. It can be administered into a vein (using a fine tube known as a cannula) or via a central (e.g. Hickman) line, by mouth, into a muscle, under the skin, or intrathecally (directly into the cerebrospinal fluid). Chemotherapy needs to be administered in ways that minimize the risks to healthy tissue, and may be given either in small doses over a long period or in high intense doses over a shorter period. It is often administered in 'blocks' of treatment, beginning with an induction phase and followed by a cycle of treatment and recovery. The short-term side effects can be unpleasant and distressing, including fever, nausea, vomiting, sore mouth, sore skin and rashes, bone-marrow suppression, and constipation. Other effects, often over a longer term, include damage to hearing, kidneys, fertility, liver, lung and heart muscle.

Radiation therapy

Radiotherapy uses high energy X-rays to destroy cancer cells. It is normally targeted specifically at the area where the tumour was found. The temporary side effects depend on the part of the body being treated, but can include sore skin, diarrhoea, loss of appetite, and nausea. The longer-term side effects can be more serious, and may have profound effects on growth and development, particularly if used in the treatment of brain tumours. Older children are less vulnerable to the adverse effects of radiation, particularly for the central nervous system, the cardiovascular system, connective tissue, and the musculoskeletal system (Bleyer 2002).

Surgery

Surgery involves cutting out the tumour, but much will depend on its size and location. It is sometimes necessary to use chemotherapy or radiotherapy to shrink the tumour before it is rendered operable. Amputation involves surgery to remove a limb in which a tumour is growing. Short-term side effects include pain at the site of the operation; longer-term effects depend on site, location and size of tumour, and the extent to which limb salvage or reconstruction is possible.

Bone-marrow and stem-cell transplantation

Bone-marrow and stem-cell transplants are ways of allowing much higher doses of chemotherapy to be given. Very high doses of chemotherapy, sometimes accompanied by radiotherapy, are given over a few days, and the destroyed bone marrow is replaced by donated bone marrow or stem cells (the child's own or a closely matched other person's). These treatments are very aggressive and would not normally be a first-line treatment.

Central venous line

Intensive chemotherapy requires good, safe access to veins for delivering the chemotherapy directly into the blood and also for obtaining blood samples for analysis. It is now standard practice for most children to have an implantable device to facilitate this process. Commonly this is a Hickman line, a synthetic soft tube inserted through the chest wall into a major blood vessel. The line can stay in for a period of months and is accessed directly for all blood sampling. An alternative device is a Portocath, a small reservoir sitting just below the skin of the chest wall and from there entering a major blood vessel. These devices require careful hygiene and are a source of infection and other complications.

Lumbar puncture

Lumbar puncture involves collection of a specimen of cerebrospinal fluid, the fluid that protects the brain and spinal cord. For younger children, lumbar punctures are usually done under general anaesthetic or sedation. For older teenagers, local anaesthetic may be sufficient. A spinal needle is inserted into the lower spinal canal and patients must lie on their side with the legs curled up to the abdomen during the procedure.

Bone-marrow aspiration and biopsy

Bone-marrow aspiration and biopsy involves an incision in the skin and insertion of needles that penetrate the bone to reach the inner core where bone marrow is produced. The marrow is withdrawn by suction or by coring out a sample of the marrow. Patients lie on their side and the procedure is usually conducted on the posterior part of the pelvic bone. It can be uncomfortable or painful and is also usually performed under general anaesthetic or sedation.

Steroids

Steroid treatment is given to children as part of the treatment to kill cancer cells, to help prevent nausea, and to reduce allergies (for example before a platelet transfusion). Side effects include irritability, increased appetite, difficulties in sleeping, and increased risk of infection.

Nutrition

The tumour, intensive chemotherapy and prolonged hospitalization all take their toll on nutrition. Many children require nutritional supplements or nasogastric feeds for periods. While negotiation about nutrition is often possible, there are situations where the medical care of the child would be compromised if advice were not followed.

Palliative care

When treatment fails, due to recurrence or progression of the tumour, a decision will be made to move to a palliative phase of treatment. Some children deteriorate and die in a short space of time, but for most children who are terminally ill the process of dying is predicted and can be planned. This involves a decision to move from an active mode of treatment to prioritizing control of symptoms. In this situation it is no longer appropriate to offer intensive treatments, and there has been a worldwide move to ensuring that most children with cancer die in their own homes with full support from hospital and community services. Each symptom is addressed its own right with consideration given to aetiology and the most effective therapy. The most commonly encountered symptoms are pain, dyspnoea (shortness of breath), nausea and vomiting, constipation, dysphagia (difficulty swallowing), agitation and seizures. Symptoms, however, vary with diagnosis. This terminal phase is usually measured in weeks.

Research on experiences of childhood cancer

The social science study of childhood cancer has been dominated by psychological studies, which have primarily identified childhood cancer as a risk to mental health and assessed its impact of the illness on the child, parents and siblings, mainly using standardized quantitative instruments. However, recent years have seen the development of a wider agenda within psychology, and the development of approaches that can more directly access the views of children themselves. At the same time, literatures from other disciplines, including anthropology, sociology, and (particularly) nursing, and using a more diverse range of methods (including qualitative approaches) are beginning to grow and contribute to our understanding of children's experiences. The value of an interdisciplinary approach is in considering these varying contributions together, rather than confining discussions within disciplinary boundaries.

This approach also demonstrates where the gaps in the research lie. The development of the literature largely reflects disciplinary preoccupations. The nursing literature, has, understandably, been focused on areas of childhood cancer experience that are open to nursing intervention, including symptom relief. Much of the qualitative research is of dubious quality, drawing very strong conclusions from very small samples, and often providing mainly descriptive rather than theoretical interpretations. What has been absent is a sustained sociological interest in the area that might illuminate the relevance of many the theoretical constructs used in explaining adults' experiences of illness.

Experiences of symptoms

Distressing symptoms (see Box 3.1) are a feature of experiences of childhood cancer, in part because of the aggressive nature of the treatments used to effect a cure. Children experience symptoms that vary over the course of illness, as well as varying in intensity. Despite the array of symptoms reported in the literature, Docherty (2003) points out that in comparison with the impressive body of research on symptom distress in adults with cancer, research on children's symptoms is much more limited. Woodgate et al. (2003) note that symptoms other than procedural-related pain and nausea and vomiting have received only minimal research attention, and that there has been an absence of research that has focused on multiple symptoms in children with cancer.

Box 3.1 Common symptoms and effects of treatment

Pain
Infection
Itchiness
Nausea and vomiting
Constipation and diarrhoea
Problems with appetite
Fatigue
Dyspnoea (shortness of breath)
Mouth problems (mucositis, mouth ulcers, and infection)
Insomnia
Irritability
Changes in appearance
Psychological distress

Symptoms are inherently subjective and in recent years there has been a welcome move towards asking children themselves about their experiences, using a range of methods including qualitative and quantitative methods. The work of Collins et al. (2000, 2002), for example, is valuable in providing information on the epidemiology of childhood cancer symptoms and in demonstrating that children are competent to provide such information without need of proxy reporting. Collins et al. (2000), in a study of 159 children with cancer aged 10 to 19, found that children can, using the Memorial Symptom Assessment Scale (MSAS), produce valid and reliable reports of their symptoms. The most common symptoms reported by children were lack of energy, pain, drowsiness, nausea, cough, lack of appetite, feeling nervous or sad, worrying, feeling irritable, itching, insomnia, dry mouth, hair loss, and vomiting. The authors emphasize that prevalence of a symptom provides little guide to severity and distress. The most distressing symptoms were reported to be difficulty in swallowing, mouth sores, pain and insomnia. Collins et al. (2002), in a later study of 189 children aged 7 to 12, found that children as young as 7 could complete a modified version of the MSAS.

A contrasting methodological approach is offered by Woodgate et al. (2003), who report a longitudinal qualitative study of 39 children and their families to explore the childhood cancer symptom courses, using methods including interviews, observations and focus groups. The meanings that children and families assigned to the symptoms were multiple and evolved as a continuous interpretive process closely associated with the meanings that children and families assigned to the overall cancer experience. When health professionals approached symptoms solely as side effects (for example, nausea), or singular physical and psychological states, children had trouble deconstructing their overall symptom experiences, including difficulties in isolating one symptom from another. Children and young people distinguished 'feeling sick' (nausea and vomiting) from 'being sick' (being unwell), and identified 'feeling yucky' as experiences that appeared to have no obvious resolution in sight. Participants also described 'feeling sore' and experiencing pain, sometimes using terms such as 'hard' pain or 'bad' pain. Symptom experiences identified as 'I feel cranky' were those experiences that caused children to feel and act differently.

Enskar et al. (1997a) also used qualitative methods in an interview-based study of 10 young people, and reported that participants found the physical side effects of treatment to be the worst aspect of having cancer, influencing their ability to live their lives the way they wanted, and causing several periods of wanting to discontinue treatments. Hedstrom et al. (2003), in a study of 50 children, 65 parents and 118 nurses, found that the most frequently mentioned aspects of distress in the physical dimension were pain resulting from diagnostic procedures and treatments, nausea and fatigue, while the most frequently mentioned aspects of distress in the emotional dimension were confinement, feeling of alienation, and worry before medical procedures.

Many symptoms may become intensified in a child who is dying. Wolfe et al. (2000) found, in a study of parents whose children who had died of cancer, that a large proportion of children were reported to have experienced a great deal of suffering in the last month of life. The percentage of children suffering from specific symptoms ranged from 19 per cent (in the case of constipation and diarrhoea) to 57 per cent (fatigue), but overall 89 per cent of children experienced 'a lot' or 'a great deal' of suffering from at least one symptom and 51 per cent from three or more symptoms. Less than 30 per cent of parents reported that the management of pain was successful, and only 10 per cent reported that nausea, vomiting or constipation were controlled.

Experiences of specific symptoms

Pain

Pain associated with disease or treatments is an important aspect of the symptom experience of children with cancer. It can be categorized into four domains depending on its aetiology (Ljungman et al. 1999):

- cancer related (for example, pain due to infiltration of the tumour in various organs or tissues);
- treatment related (for example, pain as side effects of chemotherapy and radiation);

- procedure related (for example, pain due to lumbar puncture, bone-marrow aspiration, or post-operative pain);
- pain of other aetiology.

Research thus far has been dominated mainly by psychological work with a smaller body of more qualitative research. Woodgate et al. (2003) noted that although pain scales have been valued for their clarity and simplicity and are considered useful for children with limited language skills, children in their study often became easily annoyed when asked to use them. For example, when one hospitalized 9-year-old boy was asked by his nurse to identify how 'bad' his mouth pain was by using the Wong-Baker Faces self-report scale, he hesitated and responded by stating, 'I can't use that (the scale) . . . I can't do that.' Later the child confided that he understood how to use the scale, but that he thought it was 'stupid' using it and that it just made him 'mad'. Even older children in this study did not see the merit in using self-report scales.

> Um (pause) when I was in the hospital before with my bone marrow transplant, they were always asking me to rate my pain and you can't really measure pain. So if you are feeling bad then it doesn't really matter how intense it hurts or whatever, it feels bad . . .
> (DD 16-year-old female (ALL), two years post-bone marrow transplant, quoted in Woodgate et al. 2003: 803)

Despite these problems, studies using pain-scoring systems have produced some important findings. One study examined pain in 95 children diagnosed with leukaemia for a year following diagnosis (Van Cleve et al. 2004). Average scores for pain intensity remained at or near the midpoint of the rating scales throughout the year. The most common pain sites were the legs, head/neck/abdomen and back. Pain was reported to be most intense in the morning, gradually diminishing throughout the day. Children most frequently used terms such as 'aching', 'uncomfortable', 'annoying' and 'comes and goes' to describe their pain.

Kvist et al. (1991) found that having to undergo repeated painful examinations was one of the most prominent sources of concern for children during induction therapy, while Ljungman et al. (1999) found that pain was viewed as a more troublesome symptom than nausea by most children, though there is some evidence to suggest that nausea may be a greater source of distress than pain for adolescents (Hedstrom et al. 2003). There is some evidence to suggest treatment and procedure-related pain are of greater concern to children that cancer-related pain (Ljungman et al. 1999; Van Cleve et al. 2004), but this may simply reflect the preponderance of children with leukaemia in many of the studies. Problems associated with mouth are a particular source of distress:

> When I got these side effects, sores in my throat and my mouth, and I couldn't eat. The first time it hurt so much that I couldn't sleep for a week. I was crying through the nights.
>
> (Boy, aged 11, quoted in Hedstrom et al. 2003: 126)

Pain was a common symptom for the children with cancer interviewed by Ljungman et al. (1999): 60 per cent reported pain at diagnosis, and despite subsequent treatment for pain 22 per cent reported frequent experience of moderate pain in the period after diagnosis while 7 per cent reported intense pain. More than half the children had been bedridden due to pain and 22 per cent reported not asking for pain relief because they felt that pain was an inevitable consequence of cancer, while 13 per cent did not ask because they felt nurses were too busy.

In an investigation of associations between physical pain and emotional distress, Varni et al. (2004) found that child and parent reports of pain at baseline assessment were predictive of their reports six months later, and that reports of pain and emotional distress were associated concurrently. They suggest that approaches that concentrate only on the management of pain or emotional distress are insufficient and that comprehensive, multidimensional programmes are needed to address the pain and emotional difficulties encountered by children during treatment. Research on children undergoing orthopaedic surgery for a range of different conditions has suggested that health professionals can use a range of strategies to diminish the reality or urgency of children's pain, and central to this is the prevention of children's displays of pain behaviour (Byrne et al. 2001). In view of the persistence and magnitude of pain reported by children with cancer, health professionals' strategies for managing pain would seem to warrant further study, perhaps particularly focusing on how staff respond to pain cues from children, evaluate pain and make judgements about treatment.

Fatigue

Fatigue is a defining characteristic of the experience of cancer. Recent years have seen the development of a research programme focused on issues of fatigue in children with cancer, though Erikson (2004) and Edwards et al. (2003) note a dearth of studies and a lack of direct focus on adolescents in this area. Qualitative research (Hockenberry-Eaton et al. 1998; Woodgate et al. 2003) has shown that children and young people perceive fatigue to be both physical and emotional: physical symptoms include feeling weak, sleepy, or unable to play; emotional symptoms include altered mood, not wanting to be bothered, and decrease in communication. Studies that have been conducted to date suggest that fatigue is highly subjective, holds a variety of implied meanings and associated metaphors, and can be managed by a range of coping strategies.

Some work (Davies et al. 2002) has identified energy as the core concept in descriptions of fatigue; fatigue is a dynamic, whole-person phenomenon that involves a variable flow of available energy. Children and parents distinguish between 'normal tiredness', seen as a normal and healthy process, and treatment fatigue, which is seen as unhealthy and often unanticipated. Hockenberry-Eaton et al. (1998) used focus-group interviews with samples of children and adolescents and found that adolescents described physical and mental symptoms of fatigue, including not feeling normal, feeling sorry and mad, not wanting to be bothered, feeling sleepy and wanting to lie around. Participants identified 12 causes of fatigue, including chemotherapy, the hospital environment, sleep disruptions, too many activities, boredom, fear and worry, and eight strategies to help relieve fatigue. These related to activity, rest, sleeping medication, distraction, socialization and blood transfusions. These findings were later compared with data from a study of 31 parents of children with cancer who participated in focus groups and with staff views (Hinds et al. 1999). Children and adolescents with cancer, their parents, and staff agreed on many aspects of fatigue, but they also showed subtle differences. Parents and staff viewed fatigue as a state of diminished energy. Younger children emphasized the physical dimensions of fatigue, but adolescents merged physical and mental components. Research will also need to focus on ways for managing fatigue. Davies et al. (2002), for example, showed that the noise and disruption of ward settings significantly interfered with children's ability to use fatigue-reduction strategies.

Infection

Infections are a common and virtually universal scenario linked with cancer treatment. The presence of a temperature in association with a low blood count (referred to as 'febrile neutropenia') demands an immediate response to avoid a life-threatening infection. In most paediatric studies of febrile neutropenia the mortality is now less than 1 per cent, and the improvement is solely due to early use of antibiotics and detailed attention to supportive medical care. However, experiences of fever are reported to be very distressing for children (Docherty 2003).

Psychological well-being

Studies of psychological well-being have attempted to explore psychological morbidity and maladjustment in children with cancer. Such work is important, particularly in allowing the identification of children and young people who are suffering from psychological illness that could benefit from expert intervention. However, much of the work done to date has suffered from methodological problems, and the dominance of work on psychopathology has fed a social construction of childhood cancer as a source of psychologically, as well as physically, malign processes, and has failed to illuminate other key aspects of the experience of childhood cancer.

The short- to medium-term psychological impact of childhood cancer

It is likely that some children experience intense distress in the days or weeks following diagnosis. For example, Landolt et al. (2003) found that 10 per cent of children with cancer aged 6–15 reported clinical symptoms of post-traumatic stress disorder five to six weeks after diagnosis. However, most recent studies suggest that this distress tends to resolve in the months following the diagnosis and that children with cancer do not differ from controls or population norms on most measures of psychological adjustment (Allen et al. 1997; Brown et al. 1992; Noll et al. 1999; Phipps 1999; Sawyer et al. 1997). In one of the few controlled prospective studies, Sawyer et al. (1997) assessed the psychological adjustment of 38 children at diagnosis when they were aged 2–5 years of age, and then followed these children up at one and two years after diagnosis. Immediately after diagnosis, children with cancer were reported by their mothers as more anxious, dependent, tearful, and to have more problems with sleeping than control children. However, at one and two years after diagnosis, the prevalence of problems experienced by children with cancer did not differ significantly from control children. Similarly, a UK study of 42 adolescents three weeks post diagnosis found no evidence to suggest rates of depression and anxiety were higher for children with cancer compared with controls (Allen et al. 1997). In a particularly well-conducted study, Noll et al. (1999) found that 8- to 15-year-old children currently receiving chemotherapy were similar to controls on measures of emotional well-being, and better on several dimensions of social functioning. However, there is some evidence to suggest that for older children and adolescents, the period after the end of treatment may be characterized by a higher risk of psychosocial problems than the actual treatment period itself (von Essen et al. 2000).

These findings are generally encouraging, suggesting that children and adolescents with cancer are not at elevated risk of adjustment problems during their treatment, but they also require careful interpretation. Most of the studies that have investigated this issue are small and may have insufficient power to detect small-to-moderate differences between children with cancer and controls (Noll et al. 1999). Moreover, self and parent-report instruments for measuring adjustment in children, particularly those used for measuring depression in younger children, do not achieve the levels of sensitivity and specificity of instruments used for research with adults (Sharp and Lipsky 2002). Some researchers also argue that there are particular difficulties associated with self-report instruments for measuring depression in children with cancer (Phipps 1999). It is important to note, for example, that 5–20 per cent of children and adolescents *without* cancer report significant levels of psychological distress. Therefore, any unit caring for patients within this age range is likely to encounter children who may benefit from some degree of more specialist psychological support or intervention.

Mediators of psychological impacts during treatment

Despite the lack of strong evidence to suggest that children are at substantially elevated risk of adjustment problems during treatment, a large number of studies have examined mediators of adjustment difficulties in children with cancer. Much of this work has examined associations between parental and family characteristics and the risk of psychological difficulties in children. Like much other psychosocial work on childhood cancer, a mixed pattern of results has emerged, with several studies finding associations between better child adjustment and variables such as higher family cohesion and expressiveness (Varni et al. 1996); maternal adjustment (Sawyer et al. 1998; Vance et al. 2001); maternal coping (Kupst et al. 1995) parent behaviour during medical procedures (Vance and Eiser 2004) and family socioeconomic status (Kupst et al. 1995). Other studies have found few, if any, associations between parent and family functioning and psychological outcomes in children (Kazak and Barakat 1997; Landolt et al. 2003; Stuber et al. 1996). Importantly, it is unclear how far any of the potential 'risk factors' identified are associated with clinically significant levels of maladjustment in children.

With some notable exceptions, methodological criticisms of psychosocial work on childhood cancer apply to many studies in this area, including the use of single informants of psychological adjustment (usually mothers), lack of comparison groups, small samples that cover a range of different disease and treatment types, cross-sectional designs or short-term follow-ups, and the failure to test specific hypotheses. Hill et al. (2003) make the important point that in order to investigate the role of family processes as mediators of the links between childhood cancer and adjustment difficulties it is first necessary to show that family processes are affected by childhood illness; and second, to show that these changed family processes are associated with the adjustment of family members. Yet few studies have taken this approach. Other researchers point to work suggesting that prospective associations between family functioning and child adjustment are markedly weaker than concurrent associations, and note the importance of studying adjustment changes over time (Wallander and Varni 1998). Wallander and Varni (1998) also draw attention to the wide range of factors that may mediate the relationship between paediatric chronic physical disorders and psychological adjustment. These include the nature of the disease and impairment, the degree of functional independence, the presence of other psychosocial stressors such as problems with peer relationships and friendships, and personal attributes of the child such as temperament and problem solving.

If for a moment we accept the stress/deficit model and think of childhood cancer as a risk factor for psychopathology, decades of research on developmental psychopathology examining childhood risk factors for adverse psychosocial outcomes has generated some potentially instructive observations for researchers working on psychosocial aspects of childhood cancer:

- the large magnitude of individual differences in responses to psychosocial stressors;
- the tendency for stress experiences to accentuate pre-existing characteristics or difficulties;
- the tendency for the effects of psychosocial stressors to be slight in the absence of genetic risk predispositions, but to be quite marked in the presence of such predispositions;
- multiple and long-lasting stressors are more likely to be associated with adverse outcomes that single stressors of short-duration;
- of all the environmentally mediated risks, it is exposure to the most extreme and harsh environmental difficulties (such as growing up in socially and materially impoverished institutions) that produces the most serious psychological difficulties;
- the tendency for risks of adverse psychological outcomes to be elevated for children who grow up in conditions of serious family discord and conflict, and/or who experience severely stressful life events carrying long-term threat, particularly when associated with loss or humiliation.

(Rutter 2000)

These observations point to the complexity of researching this area and the need for sophisticated research designs to unpick the complex and multiple gene-environment pathways to adverse psychosocial outcomes.

Identification of psychological morbidity is, of course, most useful if effective interventions to reduce morbidity are available. While many studies of interventions have been plagued by methodological weaknesses, there is some quite strong evidence to suggest that providing home chemotherapy for children with cancer facilitates their adjustment during the illness (Bauman et al. 1997).

More generally, the observation that concepts such as threat, loss and humiliation are important in understanding responses to stressful life events in childhood points to the need to explore the experience of cancer from the child's perspective and the meanings that it has for the child. In common with all quantitative approaches, psychological research that uses standardized instruments for understanding childhood cancer risks predetermining what is important to children and families, and excludes the possibility of other issues being discussed. Moreover, as Woodgate (2000) points out, in comparing children who have cancer with 'normal' children, it is important to avoid treating all deviations from normal as evidence of maladjustment.

Quality of life measures

Taking a broader approach than measures of psychological morbidity, measures of health-related quality of life (HRQoL) aim to offer insights into wider range domains of children's well-being. Interest in the measurement of quality of life in cancer has been sustained because of the need for measures to assess the impact of, often arduous drug and other interventions on people's well-being. However, there continues to be little agreement about the domains that should constitute the dimensions of HRQoL measures for children with cancer (Hicks et al. 2003).

Vance et al. (2001) summarize research on measuring quality of life (QoL) in childhood cancer, discussing lack of agreement about definitions of QoL and problems of measuring an essentially subjective and personally salient concept. They also point to concerns about measuring QoL in children, who may have more limited attention spans, language and reading skills, and understanding of conventional rating scales. How well-founded these concerns are is unclear, but they have led to a tendency to rely on 'proxy' reports from parents, clinical staff, or teachers. However, there is little research that has explored how proxies make their judgements, and there is growing evidence pointing to discrepancies between child and parent ratings (Eiser and Morse 2001a). Parents' reports are in fact likely to be influenced by their own mental health and their experience of stressors associated with caring. Parents do not, of course, have direct access to their children's emotional response to the illness, or to the impact it has had on their child's social life. Parents may, therefore, have different perceptions of the same situation. Where attempts have been made to explore differences between parent and child ratings, there is some evidence that parents rate their child's QoL as worse than the child does (Vance et al. 2001).

In recognition of these problems, recent years have seen the development of QoL measures aimed at assessing *both* parent proxy and child views of the child's quality of life (Varni et al. 2002). The general consensus now is that both parent and child reports of QoL are required for childhood cancer. A modular instrument, Varni et al.'s (2002) Pediatric Quality of Life Inventory (PedsQL) includes generic core scales encompassing physical functioning (8 items), emotional functioning (5 items), social functioning (5 items), and school functioning (5 items), a multidimensional fatigue scale, and a cancer module. It is available in 'developmentally appropriate' forms for ages 2–4, 5–7, 8–12, and 13–18 years. Children's self-report is measured in ages 5–18 years, and parent proxy report of child HRQoL is measured for children and adolescents ages 2–18 years. Its psychometric properties have been demonstrated to be good, and it also has the advantages of being quick and easy to complete (Eiser and Morse 2001a). In a study of survivors of childhood cancer using the PedsQL, Eiser et al. (2003) again found the mothers rated QoL as worse than the survivor, and also showed that survivors of a central nervous system tumour have worse QoL than ALL survivors. Even in ALL survivors, physical health was rated as better than psychosocial.

While measurement of quality of life will continue to have an important role, particularly perhaps in clinical trials, and while we are seeing some progress in developing instruments more sensitive to children's views and abilities, it is vital that this work is complemented by and grounded in rigorous qualitative research (Eiser and Morse 2001). The tendency to treat parents solely as proxies has also resulted in neglecting them as carers deserving of attention in their own right (Young et al. 2002), as we shall further discuss in Chapter 6.

Childhood cancer as disruption

Although symptoms are a very important part of the story of children's experiences of cancer, they are far from being the whole story. Work in the (adult) sociology of chronic illness has emphasized that the experience of illness goes well beyond the experience of symptoms. Bury (1982) proposed that chronic illness be understood as a major kind of disruptive experience, or, in Giddens's (1979) terms, a 'critical situation'. Giddens argues that a great deal can be learned about everyday situations in routine settings from analysing circumstances in which those settings are radically disturbed.

> First, there is the disruption of taken-for-granted assumptions and behaviours; the breaching of commonsense boundaries ... Second, there are more profound disruptions in explanatory systems normally used by people, such that a fundamental re-thinking of the person's biography and self-concept is involved. Third, there is the response to the disruption involving the mobilisation of resources, in facing an altered situation.
>
> (Bury 1982: 169–70).

Taking to its logical conclusion Bury's (1982) suggestion that chronic illness is precisely the kind of experience where the structures of everyday life and the forms of knowledge which underpin them are disrupted, it could be argued that study of childhood illness, including childhood cancer, could reveal much about the condition of childhood, and therefore be of great interest in terms of the theoretical development of the field of social studies of child-hood. However, there has been surprisingly little work to investigate the ex-tent to which Bury's theoretical constructs and the rich vein of subsequent research they inspired – grounded in adults' narratives of chronic illness – are useful in exploring children's and young people's experiences of cancer. Nonetheless, there is a small body of research, mostly from the nursing lit-erature, which though fragmentary and variable in quality, demonstrates some of the promise of this line of enquiry.

Disruption of social relationships

Bury's (1982) early work demonstrated the impact of chronic illness on social relationships, and in particular the disruptions of friendships and normal social activities. Maintaining normal life has to become a deliberately con-scious activity, and, for people in his study with rheumatoid arthritis, the erstwhile taken-for-granted world of everyday life becomes a burden of con-scious and deliberate action. Individuals then begin to withdraw strategically from social life, and to restrict their terrain to 'local and familiar territory' where they are least likely to be exposed to the gaze and questions of strangers and acquaintances.

Children with cancer, because of the nature of their treatment, also ex-perience massive disruption of their social relationships. For young people, the difficulty may lie in finding a context to 'be normal'. Attempts to 'pass as normal' (Goffman 1968) were prominent in Grinyer and Thomas's (2001) study of young people with cancer, but this study found that the connection to a normal life was particularly problematic during transitional stages in young adulthood, where a career has not been established and friends are moving on. A young person who is being treated around the age of 16 to 18, for example, may find that her friends have left school and are scattered around the country, or have jobs of their own.

More generally, a key difference between children and adults concerns children's obligation to return to the social world, because of the requirement that they resume school. Moreover, children are very often deprived of the adult option of returning to 'local and familiar territory', because of the re-lentless progression of the academic process: their healthy colleagues may have moved on to a different year group, sometimes even to a different school, by the time they are well enough to return to school.

There is some evidence from quantitative studies that children's friend-ships play a crucial role in their adjustment during and after chronic illness, and indeed a perceived lack of social support from classmates has been found to be one of the most consistent predictors of a range of psychological out-comes, including depression, anxiety and behaviour problems (Wallander and Varni 1998). Kameny and Bearison (2002) studied narratives of 27 young people with cancer aged between 13 and 21 years and identified severe dis-ruption to friendships among some participants:

> My friends don't come by any more, they think it's contagious.

> Last year, there was this dance at school . . . and my white count was too low to go.

> Because, actually for me I guess the hardest thing is that, is being alone.
>
> (Kamey and Bearison 2002: 161)

Studies that have investigated whether children with cancer experience more difficulties in their relationships with friends and peers have produced mixed results. Summarizing the psychological research on children's social func-tioning, Vance and Eiser (2002) outline the most popular method of assessing social relationships. This has typically involved comparison of the child with cancer with healthy control children using the Revised Class Play assessment, in which individuals are asked to imagine they are the director of a school play and must cast members of the class into appropriate roles. In some studies using this methodology, children with cancer were more often no-minated by their peers for sensitive-isolated roles (someone who is left out, whose feelings get hurt easily, or who is usually sad) than healthy control children, but children with cancer did not consider themselves to be more eligible for these roles.

Using different methodologies, other studies have found the peer group relationships among children with cancer to be severely disrupted. One study of 28 secondary schoolchildren with cancer in Finland found they were three times more likely to report having been bullied at school than sibling or peer controls (Lähteenmäki et al. 2002), though it is worth noting that the chil-dren in this study were considerably older than controls and so might be expected to have greater experience of bullying. A small qualitative study of 12 children in New Zealand (Fraser 2003) found that the effects of cancer on school friendships were, for some children, very negative, and were influ-enced by changes in the child's appearance, absences from school, mood swings, and the need to be physically treated carefully. Some children were able to maintain close friendships throughout the illness, but others had significant difficulties including stigma and rejection, and experienced social isolation, loneliness and distress.

Recent quantitative work (Noll et al. 1999), specifically designed to overcome some of the methodological difficulties of earlier studies, does not confirm these rather bleak findings, though this study focused on children who had undergone a psychosocial support programme for school re-entry, which other work has identified as successful (Wallander and Varni 1998). Reporting data from 76 children with cancer (excluding children with CNS tumours), which included ratings from matched controls and teachers as well as children with cancer, Noll et al. found no differences between cases and controls for sensitive/isolated nominations and no differences for the number of friendship nominations. Teachers selected children with cancer more often than peers for sociability-leadership roles. Children with cancer were selected less often for aggressive-disruptive roles by both peers and teachers, while loneliness scores on a range of different measures were the same for the two groups. There is some evidence that while many children with chronic illness are not at elevated risk of social problems, children who have experienced highly intensive treatment or who have central nervous system involvement in their illness may be at particular risk of difficulties (Vannatta et al. 1998a, 1998b). Nevertheless, it would seem that difficulties in social relationships are not an inevitable part of the experience of childhood cancer and that children's difficulties can be ameliorated with appropriate support.

Our small-scale qualitative study (Young et al. 2003) suggested that most children find visits by community nurses to explain the illness to classmates to be beneficial in assisting their reintegration to school. For example, several mentioned how these visits relieved them of at least some of the burden of explaining their absence. However, not all children were convinced that such interventions were helpful and a few expressed a wish to restrict which pupils were told about their illness and how much they were told.

> But then on the other side maybe it was best for me to tell them because that way I could be selective of who I told and how much I told them. Um because although – people there are a lot more mature, there are still a few prats about.
>
> (Male patient, aged 15, cited in Young et al. 2003)

One child was particularly distressed about the public way that his return to school was managed, and the exposure this gave to his illness and return to school.

> *Child:* It was quite annoying because it's embarrassing. It's alright them knowing, but my – the whole school got told once by the headmaster which was annoying. They needed to know about the [Hickman] line, but they shouldn't tell you who it is ... only your friends should know that ... all the school needs to know is that

there's a boy in it with a Hickman line so they should be more careful around everyone . . .

Interviewer: OK well that's really useful to know [child's name]. Do you think that the Macmillan nurse should ask adolescents and children who to tell at school?

Child: Just tell the teachers and I – I would tell my friends and she would have a quick word with my friends.

Interviewer: But not the whole school?

Child: No. [The nurse] had a word with the whole class and that was really annoying [unclear] that was really annoying because she went in and told the whole class and I had to show them my Hickman line, which was really annoying.

(Male patient, aged 11, quoted in Young et al. 2003)

What appears to be evident in these accounts are social aspects of the experience of childhood cancer, including stigma and shame, which have of course been persistent and helpful constructs in the sociology of (adult) health and illness (Scambler and Hopkins 1986). What is also clear is that the nature of these experiences may be quite different from those of adults, because of the way that childhood is regulated and controlled. For example, it is difficult to conceive of a situation where a public announcement, followed by a requirement to display publicly a medical device, would occur in an adult's experience of cancer.

Identity and biographical disruption

Renegotiating identity is one of the key tasks undertaken by people with cancer (Mathieson and Stam 1995). 'Identity work' is used to describe the process of patients' evaluations of the meaning of their illness within the actual context of ongoing, organized social relationships, including those with healthcare staff. It is particularly important that children's sense of identity and of 'illness' be properly understood. However, research on children's negotiations of identity has been largely lacking and is currently fragmentary.

Work to date suggests that children with cancer experience important changes in their identity, often in the form of threats. Cancer clearly threatens children's appearance, sometimes with profound implications. Kameny and Bearison's (2002) study of cancer narratives in young people reported that there was a significantly greater proportion of self-body negative statements than self-body positive statements, and participants were significantly more pessimistic when talking about their physical selves: 'Look at my leg, look at me, I'm bald and disgusting looking' (p. 159). In Dixon-Woods et al.'s (2003) study, parents reported on how the Hickman line could influence children's identity, as could scarring, amputations, and the effects of steroidal treatments. The most common threat to appearance was, of course, hair loss. This was often reported as being extremely difficult for children, especially young people, where the consequences for peer relationships and development of a romantic or sexual identity may be most keenly felt (Enskar et al. 1997a).

Children and young people may therefore engage in forms of identity work, including, as we shall describe later, concealing their illness and using strategies such as wigs to maintain a 'normal' identity. Managing issues of identity may involve significant demands on children and be a source of emotional and physical fatigue.

> She's got that whole teenage appearance thing to deal with, and just thinking about that [her possible amputation] for her has to be, has to be exhausting.
>
> (Parent, quoted in Davies et al. 2002: 15)

A number of studies describe difficulties in maintaining a socially acceptable identity among peers who do not have cancer. Bluebond-Langner et al. (1991) show how children with cancer do not feel accepted by their peers, experience ridicule, and are avoided, sometimes because cancer is perceived to be contagious. Young people in this study also reported that their healthy friends excluded them, not because they were afraid of catching cancer, but because they did not know how to act among people with cancer: 'like being kind of an outcast ... When you mention the word cancer, a lot of people just get real tight' (p. 75). The integrity of their identity was particularly threatened by the perception that they were 'different'.

Important threats to identity also arise from the dependency involved in treatment for childhood cancer. Young people appear to experience the threat cancer poses to their new-found independence most acutely, and the precarious nature of the independence at this stage of life makes it particularly difficult to give up (Grinyer and Thomas 2001; Enskar et al. 1997a). The loss of independence is especially problematic when young people need forms of care usually associated with infancy, including continence care and help with dressing (Grinyer and Thomas 2001).

Uncertainty and fear

The uncertainty, unpredictability and search for meaning associated with the outcomes of childhood cancer were highlighted by Comaroff and Maguire (1981). Woodgate and Degner (2002) identify uncertainty as one of the central experiences of childhood cancer, and Woodgate et al. (2003) described fear arising both from uncertainty *and* from anticipation. Children and young people reported being scared of forthcoming procedures, fear of death, and fear of the unknown. Hedstrom et al. (2003) similarly report fear of death and worry about procedures, describing, for example, a child aged 3 who cried as soon as he heard a noise, as he was worried somebody would come and do something to him.

Stewart (2003), in an interview-based qualitative study of 11 children with cancer aged between 9 and 12, found that children identified many examples of situations or circumstances where they experienced uncertainty. Their descriptions of uncertainty were most evident in their recollections of the initial period of diagnosis, but also occurred throughout the illness trajectory. The primary consequence of their uncertainty was negative emotional arousal, most often described as worry or fear.

Strategies, tactics and labour in childhood cancer

Aspects of normalization, coping and strategic management of chronic illness figure prominently in people's narratives of illness (Bury 2001). The literature on childhood cancer in these areas to a large extent reflects disciplinary patterns of research interest, but there is some evidence of the relevance of these constructs for children's experiences.

Coping

The concept of coping has been prominent within psychological research on adults with chronic illness, where evidence has accumulated to suggest that methods of coping that involve seeking to establish some control over the challenges posed by illness are associated with better psychological adjustment than avoidant approaches. A number of studies have also examined parents' strategies for coping with their child's illness and associations between these strategies and child and parent well-being (see, for example, Patterson et al. 2004; Sawyer et al. 1998). However, the concept of coping has not been widely used in research with children with cancer. This lack of attention probably reflects concerns with issues of development and how children's coping is largely seen as shaped by age-related factors, rather than by dispositional characteristics or situational processes (Schmidt et al. 2003).

There is some evidence that children and young people use a range of different coping strategies. Landolt et al. (2002) found that children aged between 6 and 15 (who had recently been involved in an accident or had received a recent diagnosis of cancer or diabetes) used a wide range of coping strategies, but the most common were cognitive avoidance (for example, waiting and hoping that things will get better), positive cognitive restructuring (for example reminding oneself that things will get better) and avoidant actions (such as trying to stay away from upsetting things). Some small to moderate associations were found between age and coping: younger children were found to be less likely to use active coping strategies, distraction and seeking support than older children, but there were no associations between diagnostic category or gender and children's use of coping strategies.

By contrast, a study of recent survivors of childhood cancer (Eiser et al. 2004), which explored the strategies that survivors used to deal with discrepancies between what they can and what they would like to do, found that the most commonly reported strategies involved activity changes (for example substituting an unachievable activity with a different activity), realistic plans (for example, strategies that will compensate for a particular limitation), or what the authors termed 'emotional denial' (such as reporting that a particular limitation was of little or no concern). Very few reported using strategies involving social comparison or social support. An interesting study of 84 children with cancer found that emotional adjustment was associated with positive expectations about the course of the illness and the tendency to 'deny' unpleasant emotions (Grootenhuis and Last 2001). Hinds and Martin (1988), in interviews with 58 adolescents with cancer, identify nine strategies, including distraction and looking forward, that young people use to reduce what the authors term 'cognitive discomfort'. In a smaller qualitative study of adolescents, Weekes and Kagan (1994) similarly identified strategies such as positive thinking, not thinking about treatments, keeping busy, adopting a philosophical stance and reinterpretation. Weekes et al. (1993) also found that adolescents with cancer reported that having their hand held (especially by mothers) was an effective strategy in easing treatment pain and providing reassurance. In suggesting that avoidant styles of coping may be beneficial to children, these results run counter to most reports in the adult literature.

While these studies have generated some interesting, if contradictory, findings, little is known about coping in children and about the availability of different coping strategies for children or about their changing use of coping strategies as they grow older. It is possible that concepts developed on the basis of research with adults are not applicable to children. Because children are not assigned the same autonomy as adults, they may not have the same range of strategies available to them, particularly those that involve the use of control. It is also likely that certain coping strategies or processes which are particularly important for children, for example attachment behaviours such as seeking proximity with parents, have less relevance to adults (Schmidt et al. 2003). Similarly, the mothers in our study pointed out that avoiding boredom was particularly important to children while undergoing treatment (Young et al. 2002), yet few writings on children's coping with chronic illness emphasize the importance of play or other activities. Indeed, in most taxonomies of coping, such activities are probably viewed as conceptually closest to avoidance strategies, which are usually considered to be inferior methods of coping.

It is also important to note other more general criticisms of the concept of coping and of the literature exploring associations between coping and psychological outcomes. While the original conceptualizations of coping emphasized a process which is situationally or context dependent, most research conceptualizes coping as set of static individual dispositions. Coping strategies are seen as the property of individuals rather than as a repertoire of culturally available resources for managing their experiences. For children, issues of coping need to be theorized in a much more sophisticated and sensitive way than has thus been the case, with attention given to their social positioning, agency and autonomy.

Normalization

Bury describes how normalization can involve two types of process: first where people try to 'normalize' in the sense of keeping their pre-illness lifestyle and identity intact, by maintaining usual activities and disguising or minimizing symptoms. Second, normalization can mean the redesignation of 'normal life' as containing the illness, and may involve people in signalling changes in identity rather than preserving earlier appearances. There is some fragmentary evidence of the first strategy, particularly in young people. For example, some studies have reported that older children and young people may choose to conceal their illness (for example, by non-disclosure and wearing wigs) and maintain all of their normal activities as a way of passing as normal (Rechner 1990). The evidence in the area of childhood cancer to date suggests, however, that normalization also involves the latter strategy, with a number of research reports describing the gradual development of a 'new normal'.

Clarke-Steffen's (1997) longitudinal grounded theory study of seven families of a child diagnosed with cancer with a favourable prognosis, including 7 mothers, 7 fathers, 6 ill children, and 12 siblings) emphasizes the ways in which families themselves understand and seek to manage the illness, and identified specific ways in which families operate. Though there are important limitations in her study (a homogenous small sample with similar types of cancers), she identified strategies used by families in an attempt to find a 'new normal' of predictable, reliable, comfortable routines and psychosocial contexts.

Box 3.2 Normalising childhood cancer.

Strategy	Description
Designation of normal life as containing the illness	May involve concealment of illness, and attempts to maintain normal roles and activities. For young people this might include disguise of illness using wigs, and continued attendance at education.
Designation of life with cancer as the 'new normal'	May involve dramatic changes to roles, including withdrawal from friendships and other social roles and withdrawal from education, and a discovery of new routines and roles that are now 'normal'.
Management of biographical disruption	May involve a re-thinking of future goals and aspirations, and adjustment of priorities for the future, both in the long and short-term. It may also involve profound changes to identity.
Giving meaning to illness	May involve forms attempts to answer questions such as 'why me?' 'why now?' and to link previous events to present circumstances.
Information-seeking	May involve very active forms of seeking information from books, internet, experts, support groups etc in an effort to identify what is 'normal' and what the future might hold.
Managing symptoms	The management of symptoms may become a key task that both becomes a goal and something around which a predictable 'normal' routine can be organised.

(Adapted from Clarke-Steffen 1997)

Woodgate et al. (2003) show how some symptoms also begin to be incorporated into the 'new normal'. Labelling symptoms as 'everyday' symptoms was one way for children and families to convince themselves that the children were not too sick. Children and their families to some extent could maintain a way of life similar to that pre-diagnosis, and using this strategy afforded them more control. To some extent 'everyday' symptoms became the norm:

> Like I mean things are bothering me but stomach aches and headaches, I usually don't say anything because that's normal for me now.
>
> (16-year-old female (ALL), quoted in Woodgate et al. 2003: 810)

Stewart (2003) similarly reported that children with cancer described their lives as routine, ordinary and, within the limits of an inherently unpredictable illness course, predictable. Their focus was on the routine nature of their everyday lives, and they came to feel 'ordinary' via a process they described as 'getting used to it' with the passage of time, repeated experiences, and staying flexible. 'Getting used to it' and finding the normal in the strange has been reported in a number of other studies of children's experiences of childhood cancer (Hockenberry-Eaton 1994). Stewart notes that such a finding is consistent with Davis's (1963) ethnographic study of childhood polio, in which he identified that there is an inherent orderliness in treatment regimens, and that after the crisis of diagnosis, a period of stability and order emerges with markers that point to recovery. Regaining a sense of familiarity reduces the sense of threat to the sense of being normal.

Striving for normality, then, appears to be a key task for children with cancer. This task may be easier to achieve during hospitalization, when the routines of the ward and treatments may soothe and restore a sense of inherent orderliness, and the presence of other children with the same disease will help to create peer norms. Bluebond-Langner et al.'s (1991) study of oncology camp experiences of children, for example, described the comfort involved in socializing with peers who also have cancer. Phrases used by children in this study, such as 'they can understand', 'they know how you feel' and 'you don't have to go through every single detail and explain it to them', signalled the importance of being able to be normal. Children felt less self-conscious: 'I didn't have any hair [at camp] and I didn't feel so pressured. All the kids were like me, and I didn't have to worry about the social opinion and all that jazz' (p. 74).

However, acute and potentially crisis-laden challenges to the 'new normal' arise during key transition periods, and children then assume the task of 'passing as normal'. Bluebond-Langner et al.'s (1991) work, and other research, describes the dislocation between the world of childhood cancer peers and the world outside this. For example, evidence suggests that children and young people returning to school prioritize passing as normal and seek to find ways of managing this. For the children we interviewed (Young et al. 2003), much of their talk centred on how this meant facing their altered physical and social status and encountering the responses of other children to their changed selves. They also described the burden of explanation that their illness carried, the implications of their prolonged absence for their friendships, and the restorative work they engaged in to manage their reintegration at school.

> Pretty hard actually, cause you had to get back, had to get used to the work, you had to get used to the – some of the new kids. You had to also – it's like a refreshment. It's like you're new at school . . . cause I

had to start over again with my best friends. Cause I'd been away from them so long.

> (Male patient, aged 8, quoted in Young et al. 2003)

Interviewer: What do you think when people come and ask you how you are?

Child: Um, when my friends do it – it's really annoying. They don't do it any more.

Interviewer: Don't they?

Child: No ... because I said stop asking me that.

> (Female patient, aged 12, quoted in Young et al. 2003)

The work of achieving 'normality' is thus seen as an essential part of resuming childhood, one which parents collude to produce if children themselves are unable or unwilling.

> And er initially she was very keen on going to this school because all her friends were going to the same school and she was very keen on being there and then initially she missed a few days because of going for her MRI scans and then she said she wasn't ready she didn't want to go, she just didn't want to go, she was scared ... Initially she missed a lot and we had to go on a plan because she would get up in the morning after promising the night before that she would go and normally she'd be having tears and she would have a tummy ache, sometimes I couldn't tell if it was real tummy ache or just nerves because I started getting assertive and saying look ... you have to go to school and all these things and try to be as normal as possible.
> (Mother of female, aged 11, quoted in Dixon-Woods et al. 2003: 152)

Completing therapy also functions as a key transition, one which may be experienced as something of a crisis by children as the 'normality' they have established during the treatment is no longer available. Haase and Rostad's (1994) study of seven children reported how finding out that treatment was ending could trigger a sense of confusion, followed by a period of exploring the boundaries of what completion means and seeking tangible signs of completion. They had to find a new identity and seek another 'new normal', very often very different from the normal world they left behind before they had cancer.

Strategic management

Strategic management of disease is distinguished from psychosocial issues of coping and normalization by its interest in how people mobilize resources in the wider social environment, including those from health and welfare agencies (Bury 2001). There is some fairly fragmentary evidence about children's strategic management of cancer (Hockenberry-Eaton 1994). Hockenberry-Eaton and Minick (1994), in a qualitative study of 21 children, describe how children actively participated in measures to facilitate adjustment to cancer, including engaging in distraction activities such as going for bike rides, and trying to 'get on with life'. Children described the strategic management of playing, so that they adjusted their activities to their current disease status: 'When my platelets are low, my brother just takes it easy … When my counts are up, he watches out for my central line but we can still fight' (Cody, quoted in Hockenberry-Eaton and Minick 1994: 1029).

Strategic management is likely to involve multiple negotiations between children and those caring for them. 'After my counts were okay, I got to go to a sleepover. My mom called me several times during the night, but I wouldn't come home' (girl quoted in Hicks et al. 2003: 196). These kinds of negotiation require much more exploration than they have received to date, and attention to the role of services and professional support as well as the role of parents.

The search for control

A key feature of treatment of childhood cancer is an almost complete dependence on medical technology. Without the best quality medical treatment, most children with cancer will die. Moreover, during treatment, children may also be confined to hospital for long periods of time.

Box 3.3 Ways of gaining children's cooperation

Preparing the child with information and briefing before the procedure;

play therapy and role enactments (e.g. using dolls);

pain-relieving creams;

anaesthesia;

force (e.g. parents or staff holding the child down);

bribery.

It is important here to draw attention to the highly invasive, even op-pressive nature of the treatment of childhood cancer. Treatment in most cases follows rigid protocols, which specify precisely what is to happen to the child in order to secure survival and the best long-term outcomes. In accepting the goal of survival as an outcome, parents and children must submit to these protocols; they must, in some sense, submit completely. The child's co-operation is therefore required, and where it cannot be obtained voluntarily, it may be enforced (Tomlinson 2004; see Box 3.3).

In these circumstances, it is clear that many of the recent developments in the sociology of childhood need to be rethought if they are to be applied to the particular situation of childhood cancer. Mayall's (1994a) book, for ex-ample, describes how children find themselves defined in certain ways and resist these definitions or renegotiate them. Such strategies may not be available to a child with cancer: they may find themselves defined as the objects of medical attention, and may be prevented from escaping the im-plications of this through the irresistible process of the treatment. A child in Enskar et al.'s (1997b) study illustrated this by saying, 'When taking tablets, I throw them up and I throw up each time they forced me to take them, they were very nasty' (p. 22). Similarly, Hedstrom et al. (2003) identified that children disliked physical restrictions at the hospital, being held during in-terventions, not being able to refuse treatments, and having to keep still while the drip-feed is running, but were limited in the extent that they could resist.

> And he has kicked and turned and cried and said that he doesn't want this. He knows that when he gets a needle in his implanted venous access device he gets infusions and tubes and devices. He has said many times that he doesn't want to be stuck.
> (Nurse of boy aged 4, quoted in Hedstrom et al. 203: 127)

The submission to the requirements of the medical regimen places children with cancer (and their families) in a potentially very subordinate position in relation to medical staff and organizational routines. As we discuss in Chapter 5, this has particular implications for how families communicate with staff, but it also has wider consequences for their experiences of the disease. Loss of control, including control over small, previously personal, decisions, has been identified as an important feature of adults' experiences of hospitalization (Kameny and Bearison 2002). For children with cancer, con-finement in hospital, and the invasion of privacy associated with constantly being available for intervention by staff, may be sources of strain (Hedstrom et al. 2003). Younger children may be used to sharing control over many aspects of their life with adults, but older children and young people may experience a surrender of recently-won control as deeply troubling, and may seek ways of regaining it (Kameny and Bearison 2002), potentially in highly subversive ways. The involvement of parents in aspects of life which young people consider to be their own private domain, and the vigilance of parents regarding their illness, can be very unwelcome (Weekes and Kagan 1994).

Linked to the issue of control, there has been considerable interest in issues of 'compliance' or 'adherence' with treatments for childhood cancer. There is some evidence that non-compliance is more likely in adolescents, particularly for orally-administered medications (Festa et al. 1992). Lancaster et al. (1997) investigated compliance in 496 children with 'maintenance' treatment based on anti-metabolites, an important part of treatment for ALL usually extending over two years. Nine (2 per cent) were found to have completely undetectable metabolites on more than one occasion, indicating complete non-compliance, and a further 35 had findings suggesting that they were only partially adhering to the treatment regimen. Of the nine children who were completely non-adherent, five were adolescents. A non-adherence rate of 27 per cent was found in a recent study of 44 adolescents being treated with trimethoprim/sulfamethoxazole (Kennard et al. 2004). Patients' reports of their adherence levels were found to be accurate when compared to assays of drug levels (Kennard et al. 2004). Six years after the initiation of the study, survival rates for patients categorized as non-adherent were lower than those of the adherent groups.

Emotional labour

The relevance of constructs such as emotional labour for children need to be investigated in the light of evidence suggesting that children may engage in work to protect their parents' well-being. Bluebond-Langner's (1978) classic work identifies the ceremonial orders that operate within child peer groups in relation to dying. She found that children quickly learn that death is an inappropriate topic for conversation with adults, and is instead something to be discussed in peer groups only. Her study demonstrates that children know much about their illness without ever being told directly, and may engage in what she calls 'mutual pretence': an unvoiced agreement that prognosis will not be discussed. She found that this strategy is the dominant mode of interaction between terminally ill children and those who care for them, and can be interpreted as a collusion to protect hope. The finding that children engage in emotional labour to protect their parents' well-being has been found in some other studies, as have the consequences for children's own well-being (Stewart 2003).

Conclusions

Study of experiences of childhood cancer has long been dominated by the psycho-oncology approach, which has remained preoccupied with the identification of psychological morbidities and processes of adjustment and adaptation. Such an approach is clearly important, but is very far from being the whole story. A key problem has been its tendency to represent children and young people as passive victims of malign processes, and its failure to explore the ways in which children and young people give meaning to their experiences. A smaller body of work, mainly using qualitative methods, has begun to redress this problem and reveal some of the ways in which children with cancer function as agents and are active in forging meaning.

This qualitative work, though of variable quality, suggests that many of the constructs that have been developed in the sociology of adult chronic illness help to explain the ways in which children and young people negotiate cancer. There is, for example, evidence that cancer is experienced as disruption and a threat to a taken-for-granted world, with effects including biographical disruption, altered identity and social relationships; and that children and young people engage in active forms of coping (though perhaps not as conventionally theorized within adult psychology), strategic management of the illness, normalization, and other forms of work related to their cancer. Events which initially appear to defy absorption into everyday routines (Giddens 1991) become challenges to which children have to rise. Switches between home and hospital worlds may, for example, require a range of different strategies from children and young people and involve various forms of labour, including identity work. This agentic conceptualization of children's experiences is, of course, consistent with the position we adopted at the outset of this book and with the theorization of agency in the 'new' social studies of childhood. However, there is some evidence that aspects of the ways in which children and young people characteristically negotiate cancer are age related. For example, the impact on identity and social relationships may be much more powerful in older children and young people, but may be of little significance to younger children.

What is also evident is that the repertoire of strategies available to children, and the extent to which they can assert control over the work they do in relation to their cancer, may differ in fundamental ways from those of adults. Some repertoires are more available to children – for example kicking and screaming at the prospect of an intervention – but children may also find themselves much less able to resist things they do not want, and may be much more constrained in their ability to function autonomously. In managing their altered identity and attempts to pass as normal, for example, children and young people have to negotiate the relentless progression of school life, and may be unable to use strategies familiar to adults, such as withdrawal. The public aspects of childhood cancer, and the extent to which young people who experience it are under surveillance and control, makes their experience of illness distinctive from that of adults. In other respects, however, children and young people may be able to assert more or less concealed forms of autonomy, for example through a 'secret' assumption of responsibility for emotional labour, or through non-adherence, particularly in young people.

It is clear that more work will need to be done on the methods for exploring children's experiences of cancer. Much of the theorizing in the sociology of adult chronic illness has been based on illness narratives, which take characteristic forms and have distinctive features (Bury 1982; Hyden 1997). The extent to which children's and young people's narratives of cancer are distinctive from those of adults, including the extent to which these narratives vary by age, has remained under-explored. The potential for ethnographic work has also remained under-realized.

4   Late effects of childhood cancer

Rapid improvements in the treatment and survival of children with cancer were first realized in the 1970s, and the first large cohort of survivors of childhood cancer is now progressing through adulthood. Already it is estimated that 1 in 1000 adults aged between 20 and 29 years is a survivor of childhood cancer and the number of long-term survivors will increase substantially in the coming decades (see Figure 4.1).

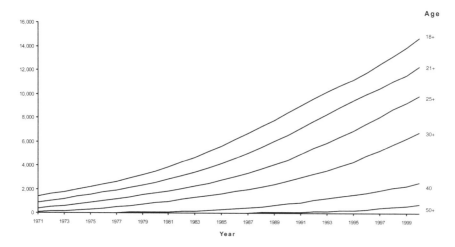

Figure 4.1 Adult survivors by age group in the UK.

Source: National Statistics Website: www.statistics.gov.uk
Crown copyright material is reproduced with the permission of the Controller of HMSO

The treatment responsible for improved survival also produces a range of adverse long-term consequences that may limit survival duration and have a range of other impacts. These adverse long-term health-related outcomes are commonly referred to as 'late effects' of childhood cancer. Late effects are varied, with considerable variations according to the cohort studied, the primary disease, treatment and host-related factors (Friedman and Meadows 2002). In a review of a regional follow-up service in the UK, 58 per cent of survivors were found to have at least one 'chronic medical problem' and 32 per cent had two or more (Stevens et al. 1998).

There are a large number of potential late effects; and they can be broadly divided into organ dysfunction, second malignant neoplasm, early mortality, decreased fertility and adverse neurocognitive sequelae. A parallel body of work has begun to document the psychosocial and psychopathological late effects of childhood cancer. To an even greater extent than the literature on experiences of childhood cancer, study of the experiences of late effects has been dominated by psychological approaches, and has used a psychopathological or deficit model that, we will argue, is less than adequate for understanding the experiences of the majority of childhood cancer survivors.

Physical and neurocognitive late effects

The factors contributing to the late effects include surgery, radiotherapy and chemotherapy treatments as well as underlying genetic and biological factors (Tables 1 and 2).

Radiotherapy

Radiotherapy directly damages cancer cells as well as normal tissues within the radiation field. Late effects are therefore related anatomically to the site of the radiotherapy field as well as the dose of radiotherapy given.

Chemotherapy

Chemotherapy prevents cancer cells dividing and surviving. Although cancer cells are most sensitive to chemotherapy, normal tissues are also affected. Specific chemotherapy drugs will affect a range of organs of the body and the pattern of potential damage varies depending on the combination of drugs being used.

Fertility

Radiotherapy and chemotherapy can both affect fertility, though recent years have seen a movement towards attempting to preserve fertility through sperm-banking (for post-pubescent males) and collection and storage of ovarian tissue, though this latter is currently still in a developmental stage.

If the ovaries or testes are in the radiation field, patients are liable to be rendered infertile. Radiotherapy to the brain may result in reduced hormonal secretions from the pituitary-hypothalamic axis, which may impact on fertility, although it is usually possible to treat this with replacement hormones. Commonly used drugs in chemotherapy cause direct toxicity to the gonads.

Table 4.1 General guidelines for common radiation late effects assessment and management

System	Potential effects	Monitoring guidelines
Central nervous system	Precocious puberty, growth hormone deficiency, other hormonal deficiencies, cognitive dysfunction, hearing loss	Endocrine monitoring, including growth and gonadal status Neurocognitive testing Hearing tests
Eye	Cataracts	Eye examination
Cardiac	Cardiomyopathy (muscle weakness) Coronary artery disease	ECG, echocardiogram
Lung	Pulmonary fibrosis	Lung function tests
Thyroid gland	Hypothyroidism Thyroid cancer	Thyroid function tests
Gonadal	Ovarian failure Oligospermia	Hormone analysis
Second malignancies	Sarcoma, CNS tumours, breast cancer, melanoma, others.	Regular examination (annual)
Organs	Any organ within the field of radiation may sustain dysfunction, or be at risk for development of a second cancer	

(Adapted from Friedman and Meadows 2002)

Fertility deficits vary with the age at time of treatment, the type of treatment and the site of treatment. Since the majority of childhood cancers occur at a young age, a long period of follow-up is required and present studies reflect the treatment protocols in use 20 years ago. A Norwegian study of acute lymphoblastic leukaemia (ALL) survivors reported that the first successfully treated generation of females had a nearly normal reproductive pattern during young adulthood, without increased risk of congenital anomalies in the offspring (Nygaard et al. 1991). Survivors who had received prophylactic radiation of the central nervous system had a lower first birth rate than those without radiation. In more recent years radiotherapy for ALL has been removed for the majority of patients and the infertility risk would be classed as 'low'.

In contrast, treatment of Hodgkin's disease is known to produce significant deficits in fertility, with males most susceptible. Mackie et al. (1996)

Table 4.2 General guidelines for common chemotherapy late effects assessment and management

System	Agent	Potential effects	Monitoring guidelines
Central nervous system	Intrathecal methotrexate	Cognitive dysfunction	Neurocognitive evaluation
Hearing	Platinum drugs	Hearing loss	Audiology evaluation
Cardiac	Anthracyclines	Cardiomyopathy	ECG, echocardiogram
		Arrhythias	
Lung	Bleomycin	Restrictive lung disease	Lung function tests
Liver	Methotrexate	Liver dysfunction	Liver function tests
	Thioguanine		
	Mercaptourine		
	Actinomycin		
Kidney	Platinum drugs	Renal insufficiency	Kidney function test, urine analysis
	Alkylating agents		
Gonadal	Alkylating agents Nitosureas	Ovarian failure Early menopause	Hormonal analysis Reproductive counselling
		Testicular failure	
Second malignancy	Alkylating agents	Leukaemia	Blood count
	Platinum drugs		Examination
	Topoisomerase inhibitors		

(Adapted from Friedman and Meadows 2002)

reported that up to 89 per cent of males treated before puberty have been reported to have evidence of severe damage to the testes, resulting in permanent infertility. Around 50 per cent of girls treated prepubertally with six or more courses of chemotherapy had evidence of subtle ovarian damage. The authors comment that further follow-up is required to determine if these women have recovery of function or go on to develop premature menopause (Mackie et al. 1996).

Table 4.3 Risk of future fertility compromise associated with different childhood cancers

Low	Medium	High
Acute lymphatic leukaemia	Acute myeloid leukaemia	High-dose chemotherapy
Localized tumours of muscles	Wilm's tumour	Bone marrow transplant
Brain tumour requiring surgery only	Bone tumour (osteosarcoma)	Bone tumour (Ewing's sarcoma)
	Neuroblastoma	Hodgkin's Disease
	Soft tissue sarcoma	(alkylating-based therapy in males)
	Non-Hodgkin's lymphoma	Soft tissue sarcoma – metastatic
	Hodgkin's disease (depends on protocol)	
	Brain tumour	

(Adapted from: A strategy for fertility services for survivors of childhood cancer. By a Multidisciplinary Working Group convened by the British Fertility Society. See: www.fertility.org.uk/practicepolicy/)

Second malignancies

The treatment used for cancer can in itself damage normal cells, which over a period of time can develop into secondary, and otherwise unrelated, cancer. The cumulative risk for developing a second malignant tumour at 20 years after completion of cancer treatment is 5 to 20 times greater than that expected in the general population. Both radiotherapy and certain chemotherapy drugs are implicated. Once again certain subgroups appear to be at greatest risk. For example, children with Hodgkin's disease treated with a combination of radiotherapy and chemotherapy are at high risk with a cumulative incidence of a second malignant tumour at 30 years of 26 per cent (Green et al. 2000). The most frequent second cancers are thyroid, breast, skin cancer, Non-Hodgkin's lymphoma and leukaemia.

Neurocognitive effects

Neurocognitive effects are most evident for patients treated for brain tumours (Mulhern et al. 2004). Many survivors of brain tumours have had surgery and radiotherapy, both of which are damaging to the developing brain and most damaging to very young children. The reduction in non-verbal and information processing skills is most prominent with deficits in short-term memory, visual motor integration, sequencing and attention and con- centration being most common. Even with help, survivors of brain tumours have been found to have a low educational achievement with employment rates as low as 50 per cent (Hays 1993). Smaller, but still important neuro- cognitive effects have been shown for other tumour groups, including acute leukaemia, where treatment is given to prevent infiltration of the central nervous system by leukaemia cells.

Psychological morbidity

The study of psychosocial late effects has been dominated by studies of psy- chological morbidity. Several studies suggest that the self-esteem of survivors is unaffected (Evans and Radford 1995; Felder-Puig et al. 1998; Langeveld et al., 2004) or even improved (Anholt et al. 1993; Gray et al. 1992) by the experience of childhood cancer.

By contrast, findings on rates of depression and anxiety in survivors have tended to be quite inconsistent over the last few decades. Results of studies conducted before the 1990s suggested that survivors were at considerable risk of adverse psychological outcomes. Lansky et al. (1986) regarded survivors as having an interruption in their development, which they are unable to overcome, while Koocher and O'Malley (1981) reported adjustment problems in 59 per cent of the survivors they studied. They characterized experiences of survivorship as the 'Damocles Syndome' to refer to the persistent underlying anxiety about disease recurrence, body image, and long-term effects of treatment felt by survivors and their families. This contrasts with the findings of studies conducted during the 1990s, which have produced little or no evidence of elevated risks of depression or anxiety-related disorders in survi- vors (Mackie et al. 2000; Stam et al. 2001). A systematic review of studies published between 1990 and 1998 found little evidence to suggest that sur- vivors experience lasting difficulties: of the 13 studies which examined ad- justment, anxiety or depression, nine reported no differences between survivors and controls or population norms, two reported more psychological difficulties in survivors, while two suggested that survivors experience fewer psychological difficulties (Eiser et al. 2000b). Most of the studies available for this review used instruments that were questionnaire-based and that only assessed current functioning, but a well-conducted study that used standar- dized diagnostic interviews, which allow assessment of problem severity over specific time periods, also found no evidence of elevated rates of major or minor depression in survivors compared with unrelated controls (Mackie et al. 2000). There was also no difference in the numbers of survivors and controls who had had any psychiatric disorder.

It is difficult to account for the inconsistencies in studies conducted be- fore and after 1990, but the bleak picture for survivors in the pre-1990 studies may be an artefact of sampling and measurement difficulties. It could also point to treatment differences over the decades, or to the inadequacies of psychosocial care for families in earlier decades. More recently, two very large scale multi-centre studies of long term survivorship have produced consistent results suggesting that survivors are at moderately greater risk of psychological distress than in their siblings (Hudson et al. 2003; Zebrack et al. 2002b). This suggests that studies conducted in the 1990s, which typically had sample sizes of 100 or fewer, were under-powered to detect moderate effect sizes.

One of these studies examined the health status of 9535 individuals who had been diagnosed with a range of different types of cancer, and 2916 of their siblings (Hudson et al. 2003), using a self-report mental health screening tool specifically devised for use with cancer patients. Survivors were found to be 1.8 times more likely to report mental health problems than siblings. The percentage of all survivors estimated to be experiencing mental health problems was 17.2 per cent compared with 10.2 per cent of siblings. This is substantially higher than that found by Zebrack et al. (2002b), a difference that is probably due to the sampling and measurement differences between the two studies, including Hudson's use of a less conservative screening tool to estimate mental health difficulties. Nevertheless, it is striking that these two studies produce odds ratios that are broadly comparable and that both studies are consistent in suggesting that survivors have a moderately elevated risk of psychological distress compared with their siblings. However, Zebrack et al. (2003: 1455) concludes that the 'most potent finding is the low level of psychological symptomatology' among survivors.

While there is good reason to have confidence in the results of these very well-conducted and large-scale studies, it should be noted that both used sibling control groups, which may lead to the under-estimation of the psychosocial late effects for survivors of childhood cancer (Cuttini et al. 2003). Siblings of childhood cancer survivors share some of the difficulties of their brother or sister's illness and may be at elevated risk of adverse psychological outcomes. The alternative possibility of using unrelated controls is not without its problems either, since such studies cannot control for possible environmental and genetic differences between cases and controls.

It should also be noted that neither of these large-scale studies used a standardized diagnostic measure of psychological morbidity so it is difficult to draw conclusions about the severity of the difficulties experienced by survivors who reported psychological distress. A recently published study of rates of psychiatric hospitalizations between 1970 and 1993 among 3710 survivors found the risk of hospitalization for psychiatric disorder is not increased among survivors, with the exception of survivors of brain tumour (Ross et al. 2003). This suggests that if survivors experience psychiatric difficulties, in most cases these are not sufficiently severe to warrant hospitalization.

There is some evidence that certain sub-groups of survivors are at heightened risk of severe psychiatric difficulties. Survivors who have had a brain tumour have a greater risk of hospitalization for a psychiatric complaint compared with the general population, and a substantially greater risk for hospitalization for psychoses of somatic, cerebral causes (Ross et al. 2003). Evidence that brain tumour survivors are at a particularly high risk of disorders with a somatic component indicates that biological rather than psychological factors may be involved mediating risk of some forms of psychoses. Importantly, Ross et al. (2003) found no evidence of increased risk of hospitalization for affective disorders such as major depression among survivors as a whole, or for survivors of brain tumours.

Risk factors for psychological morbidity

A wide range of risk factors for anxiety and depression in survivors has been postulated, but evidence for many of these is contradictory (Stam et al. 2001). These inconsistencies are partly attributable to the tendency of many studies in psychosocial oncology to be small-scale, and to the lack of capacity to investigate disease and treatment-specific effects. Based on the large-scale studies reviewed above, a pattern is emerging to suggest that the following factors may place survivors at increased risk of mental health difficulties:

- Demographic factors: low socio-economic status; female gender; lower educational attainment; low income (Hudson et al. 2003; Zebrack et al. 2002b)
- Disease factors: central nervous system tumours (Langeveld et al. 2003; Zebrack et al. 2002b) Hodgkin's disease, sarcoma, bone tumour, second malignant primary cancer (Hudson et al. 2003)
- Treatment factors: exposure to intensive chemotherapy (Zebrack et al. 2002b) cranial radiation therapy (Haupt et al. 1994; Pui et al. 2003)

Other risk factors for anxiety and depression have long been postulated, but Zebrack et al. (2002b) found no evidence to suggest that age at diagnosis, time since diagnosis, or duration of treatment were associated with risk of psychological distress and Hudson et al. (2003) found no evidence to suggest that ethnic minority status or era of diagnosis was associated with mental health difficulties.

Care and treatment of late effects

Recent attention has focused on the 'surveillance' of survivors of cancer, with the aim of improving knowledge of the risks and causes of late effects in order to inform and refine treatments for subsequent generations of childhood cancer survivors (Wallace et al. 2001). Follow-up surveillance may also confer some advantages to individual survivors, including evaluation of potentially significant symptoms, medical care for managing or ameliorating late effects, reassurance that their health is being monitored, and providing information about the illness, its treatment and implications (Institute of Medicine 2003). Such information is likely to be of considerable importance in managing the late effects of treatment and in dealing with possible misconceptions about the illness.

There is, of course, a tension between ensuring that survivors have access to appropriate information while avoiding exposing them to any that induces or adds to the sense of uncertainty and vulnerability that surrounds survivorship. One unfortunate outcome of an intervention designed to enhance survivors' awareness of the importance of follow-up and the need for vigilance about their health was an increased sense of vulnerability to future health problems (Eiser et al. 2000b).

Researchers might also turn their attention to the potential consequences of this surveillance, which concentrates on identifying the particular 'deficits' in children and their families, while rather less attention is given to how services could better support survivors. Particularly worrying is the lack of evidence for many psychosocial interventions that have now become routine and unquestioned aspects of clinical practice (Bauman et al. 1997). The potential for iatrogenic harm that might be associated with some of these interventions is rarely discussed in the literature, let alone questions about the acceptability or experiences of these interventions. This is particularly important in view of how little note has been taken of how children with cancer and their families conceptualize their needs and their situation. It is remarkable, for example, how little we know about how survivors themselves construct their experience of illness, the processes of adaptation to illness and what forms of psychological or other support is likely to helpful to them in this process.

Late effects as survivorship

In Chapter 3 we showed that study of the symptoms of childhood cancer provides only partial insight into the experiences. Similarly, study of the physical and psychosocial 'late effects' of surviving childhood cancer provides only a limited account. Experiences of childhood cancer survival would appear to be well suited to a narrative-based approach that could go beyond the static identification of things that go 'wrong'. Recent years have seen the emergence of a small body of research using qualitative methods to study the experiences of survivors. Again, like the literature on having childhood cancer, this has been helpful and promising, but much of the work (with some important exceptions) is beset by methodological problems and there is a tendency towards description rather than theorization.

Two useful approaches to theorization can be identified, the first within the sociology of chronic illness, and the second (to some extent a subsidiary literature) within the study of survivorship. In Chapter 3 we outlined how the sociology of chronic illness has understood the experience of illness as a major form of disruption with widespread social and biographical effects, and provoking a range of responses (Bury 1982). Such an approach would appear to be full of potential for exploring the late effects of childhood cancer, but very little research has been conducted which has adopted non-deficit models to understand the experiences of survivors. Even research on coping, which is sometimes presented as embodying an approach that avoids understanding individuals' experiences in terms of psychopathology, is still largely concerned with deficits in survivors or families' strategies for dealing with their experiences (Parry 2003). These allow only limited insight into how individuals themselves understand, construct or represent their experiences, though it is possible to identify how some of the work can help to inform an understanding of late effects as disruption. There is, moreover, a need to distinguish, conceptually, different forms of 'late effects'. Some late effects constitute new forms of chronic illness in their own right (for example new malignancies) while others are impairments or disabilities (for example, cognitive and fertility impairments). Some late effects are secondary to these illnesses or impairments, but other late effects will be produced by the original disease and the experience of that disease.

The literature on survivorship in cancer is relatively recent, but very promising. Little et al.'s (2002) work on survivorship and discourses of identity, though not directly addressing issues of childhood cancer, is very useful in helping to theorize the field. Drew's (2003) study of self-reconstruction and biographical revisioning following cancer in childhood or adolescence is an important empirical and theoretical move forward within the specific field of childhood cancer. Both of these studies themselves utilize theory and concepts developed by Frank (1995). Drawing on this work, in the following sections we organize the material using some of the constructs that we believe may be useful in understanding experiences of childhood cancer late effects. The primary material on which we draw is not, for the most part, itself organized in this way.

Experiences of survivorship and the social construction of survivorship

Drew (2003) argues that, contrary to the modernist position of biomedicine, which sees people as either sick or well, the notion of 'cure' is problematic in relation to childhood cancer. There is, therefore, little possibility of 'owning' a tidy ending for people who have experienced this disease. Indeed, Frank

(1995) proposes that experience of serious illness can be understood as analogous to social characteristics such as 'ethnicity' in terms of their implications for an irrevocable, albeit negotiated, identity. Little et al. (2000), with reference to adult cancer survivors, describe this as the peculiar adhesiveness of the cancer diagnosis, while Stacey (1997) points to the lack of a script for a complete resolution of a cancer experience of disturbance, of temporality and self-perception. Drew's (2003) work graphically illustrates this, showing how some participants in her study resented their cancer survivorship as a master status. She gives the example of Alice, who won a Rhodes scholarship:

> The headline of pretty much every article was, you know – 'cancer survivor' or 'Rhodes winner lucky to be alive' … I've found it really annoying that everyone – every article capitalized on that … I think to a certain extent I felt this sort of devalues my achievement, you know.
>
> (quoted in Drew 2003: 189)

Drew (2003) promotes the idea that a useful way forward can be found in the theoretical construct of 'biographical revisioning', where people circumvent or reinvent taken-for-granted social assumptions about their illness trajectory and find new ways to repair ruptures between self, body, and society. She proposes that survivors develop a 'consciousness of survival', and argues that there is a need to understand the efforts of survivors in reworking and working within and around dominant cultural constructions of their illness experience.

The importance of this insight is illustrated by the literature on adult survivors of cancer, which alerts us to the narrow range of socially acceptable positions that survivors can adopt on their experiences, and the lack of suitable discourses for representing their experiences (Little et al. 2002). For adult survivors, the negotiation of social constructions of survivorship may involve very active forms of labour and severely limit what is socially possible. Little et al. (2002) argue that survivors can 'fit only into pre-existent and inadequate paradigms of the normal or the chronically ill, into metaphors of the victim or the hero'. Stacey (1997), for example, in her critique of cancer narratives, shows how most narratives emphasize the heroic qualities demanded of the cancer patients.

In Drew's (2003) study, there was evidence in some accounts of survivors of childhood cancer of resistance to the imposition of the 'hero' narrative, and a preference for a less demanding social position:

> One thing I wish [my doctors] would've done at the time – to mention that there would be recovery time … when I'd go back, it was always 'you look so well', or 'you're so lucky' and I couldn't say

'well actually I don't feel lucky' because after everything they'd done
for me, I felt like I didn't appreciate it.

(quoted in Drew 2003: 190)

We would argue that in most cases it might be more helpful to see this
not as evidence of individual psychopathology or inefficient coping, but as an
indication of the lack of cultural repertoires for representing the experience of
survivorship and of the social sanctions that might be applied to those whose
accounts of survival display unresolved tensions and difficulties (Little et al.
2002; Little and Sayers 2004). Little et al. (2002) argue that what is needed is a
discourse which acknowledges that survivorship is a life lived in a context of
new knowledge, and that recognizes both the continuity of identity and the
powerful forces of change inherent in the extreme experience.

This kind of theorization is important in explaining some of the findings
from the psychological literature, which have indicated that some self-
reported psychosocial outcomes for survivors are comparable to, or only
moderately worse than, comparison groups. These findings have led some
researchers to discuss the possibility that positive outcomes for survivors may
be explained by processes such as denial or 'response shifts' (Langeveld et al.
2004; Stam et al. 2001). Response shift theory suggests that the experience of
life-changing events such as childhood cancer may result in a downward
calibration of people's internal standards for evaluating or conceptualizing
their lives (Schwartz et al. 1999).

Response shift theory has parallels with debates about the so-called
'disability paradox', whereby chronically-ill or disabled individuals generally
rate the value of their lives more highly than non-disabled individuals who
imagine themselves with a chronic illness or impairment (Albrecht and
Devlieger 1999). However, it has been argued that application of the term
'paradox' to this phenomenon is inappropriate, since it rests on the mistaken
assumption that deviation from physical normalcy produced by a physical
impairment must diminish quality of life (Koch 2000).

Along with many theorists, we would agree that individuals who have
lived through an extreme experience such as life-threatening illness may
undergo a process of revaluation or reprioritization akin to a response shift,
and Drew's (2003) narrative analysis provides some support for this. However,
we would argue that where this results in ratings from survivors that are
broadly equivalent to those of the general population, in most cases this
represents a largely life-enhancing process of revaluation. To label it as a form
of denial, beneath the surface of which must lie some adjustment problems,
seems to misappropriate or devalue this process and the reordered meanings
that survivors may construct to understand their experiences. The discourse
of disbelief or distrust that seems to accompany some discussions of self-
report data from survivors therefore seems unfortunate and unwarranted.

This context is important in interpreting the few qualitative studies that have been conducted on the experiences of survivors of childhood cancer (Karian et al. 1998; Lozowski 1993; Parry 2003). All these studies point to the positive aspects of survivorship, including the ways in which the experience of survivorship can reaffirm the value of life, and the confidence and strength that some survivors derive from the knowledge that they have survived. Two of these studies also deal with the worries and uncertainties that are present in the accounts of survivors (Lozowski 1993; Parry 2003). For example, Parry notes that uncertainty had become part of the landscape of the lives of all survivors in her study, but for most it was no longer experienced as solely distressing, nor did it require active management; rather, participants' accounts revealed how uncertainty acted as a catalyst to revaluate their priorities, brought a deep appreciation of life, and a stronger sense of confidence, resilience and optimism. Uncertainty had a transformational potential: by becoming more aware of the uncertainties of life, survivors were able to value life more fully. The authors of these studies contemplate the possibility that survivors' accounts of the gains brought about by their illness were shaped by processes of denial or avoidant coping. However, they dismiss this explanation, commenting that the depth and coherence of survivors' accounts is not consistent with denial. Similarly, other researchers show how a positive orientation to life can coexist with quite substantial worry (Zebrack and Chesler 2001). Although we cannot discount these observations about the positive outlook of survivors, the particular status of survivorship, as already discussed, must rest as an explanation for these findings.

Importantly, Drew's (2003) work also cautions against seeing late effects as the kinds of static outcomes that they are sometimes characterized as by the quantitative literature. She emphasizes the need to see survival as a multifaceted, dynamic, ongoing process involving a biographical revisioning and self-reconstruction. People incorporate an illness history into their identity, but others may experience illness in such a way that they do not accommodate the illness history, making identity work very complex. In most cases, however, survival continues a process of self-reconstruction, involving activities and introspection and examination of personal narrative. This is evident, for example, in Drew's reports concerning childhood cancer survivors' narratives about fertility, which demonstrate how people may have to deal with the potentially unsatisfactory consequences of survival. She notes that motherhood was more likely to appear in these narratives as a key feature of self-concept and imagined social role than fatherhood, illustrating the potentially gendered nature of survivorship processes.

Disruption of social relationships

In Chapter 3 we showed that disruption of social relationships is an almost inevitable feature of childhood cancer, and that issues of identity and normalization are important to children and young people with cancer. Several studies, conducted mainly within the psychology paradigm, suggest that survivors of childhood cancer may experience problems with social functioning (Eiser et al. 2000b). Mackie et al. (2000) reported that 30 per cent of cancer survivors were assessed as having a combination of difficult love/sex relationships and friendships compared to only 5 per cent of controls. Cancer survivors were also more likely to be assessed as displaying avoidant functioning in love/sex relationships, indicating that they had shorter relationships or relationships characterized by lack of involvement, compared with controls. However, there were no differences between survivors and controls in rates of avoidant functioning for friendships and non-specific social contacts. In addition, there were no differences for cancer survivors and controls on measures of their *current* social functioning.

While other studies have found no evidence of difficulties in the social functioning of survivors (Madan-Swain et al. 1994; Noll et al. 1993; Pendley et al. 1997), at present the balance of evidence suggests that some survivors may struggle with aspects of their social lives (Stam et al. 2001). However, definitive large-scale studies on social functioning of the sort that have recently been published on the mental health of survivors have yet to be conducted. Interestingly, there is some evidence that an intensive and well coordinated programme of support may minimize problems with social functioning (Reiter-Purtill et al. 2003), indicating that difficulties for survivors of childhood cancer may not be inevitable.

Biographical disruption: intimate relationships, education and employment

Several studies suggest that childhood cancer survivors are less likely to form and maintain long-term intimate relationship and to get married than peers (Byrne 1989; Green et al. 1991; Langeveld et al. 2003; Pui et al. 2003). However, it is likely that many of these differences are attributable to low rates of marriage among certain sub-groups of survivors, particularly survivors of central nervous system tumours and those who have experienced neurotoxic forms of treatment, and that other groups of survivors have rates comparable to those of siblings or the general population (Byrne 1989). A recent study of survivors of acute lymphoblastic leukaemia, all of whom were at least 10 years post-treatment, found that rates of marriage in survivors who had not been treated with cranial radiation were comparable to the general population (Pui et al. 2003). However, 35 per cent of women who had undergone cranial radiation therapy had married, compared with 48 per cent of women who had not undergone cranial radiation therapy. These researchers have suggested that this finding is consistent with the greater vulnerability of women to the physiological effects of cranial radiation therapy (Pui et al. 2003).

It also appears that some survivors are at greater risk of poorer educational and employment outcomes than controls (Green et al. 1991; Haupt et al. 1994; Langeveld et al. 2003; Mitby et al. 2003; Pui et al. 2003), findings which are to be expected given the well-documented neurotoxic effects of many treatments for childhood cancer and the disrupting effects of the disease and treatment on children's education. Again, however, it seems that this risk varies widely among different diagnostic and treatment sub-groups. For example, one study found that survivors of ALL were more likely to need special education services, and that those who had received the highest doses of cranial radiation therapy were the most likely to use these services and least likely to enter college. However, survivors as a whole were just as likely as their siblings to enter college and graduate, indicating that with appropriate educational support most were eventually able to overcome the difficulties presented by their illness and treatment (Haupt et al. 1994). Similar findings were observed in a recent study of the educational attainment of 12,430 survivors (Mitby et al. 2003). In particular, survivors of leukaemia central nervous system tumours, non-Hodgkin's lymphoma and neuroblastoma were significantly less likely to complete high school compared with siblings. But when they received appropriate special education support, most survivors were just as likely to complete high school as their siblings. The only exception to this were survivors of central nervous system tumours and kidney tumours.

In the light of the impact of some forms of childhood cancer and treatment on educational attainment, it is also not surprising that some survivors are less likely to be employed than their peers. For example, one study found that while the rates of employment among survivors of acute lymphoblastic leukaemia who had not received cranial radiation therapy were comparable to population norms, men and women who had been treated were, respectively, almost three and seven times more likely to be unemployed than the general population (Pui et al. 2003).

Taken as a whole, these findings suggest that most survivors overcome the difficulties associated with their disease and treatment and achieve relationship, educational and employment outcomes comparable to those of sibling comparison groups and population norms. Special educational provision is likely to be of great importance in enhancing the educational and employment outcomes of survivors and helping them to overcome the difficulties associated with their illness and treatment. However, survivors who have had central nervous system involvement in their disease or treatment remain at risk of a range of poor outcomes.

Fear and uncertainty

Drew's (2003) study of childhood cancer survivors' narratives shows how uncertainty and unpredictability are central features of their experiences. This finding is confirmed by quantitative research. In one large-scale study 13 per cent of survivors reported moderate to high levels of concern about cancer-specific issues (Hudson et al. 2003). Those who had been diagnosed with Hodgkin's disease, sarcomas and bone tumours were more likely to report cancer-related fears and anxieties than other survivors.

Evidence also suggests that survivors worry less about general health issues than comparison groups, but they worry more about cancer-specific issues (Lozowski 1993; Weigers et al. 1998; Langeveld et al. 2004). One study of 400 long-term survivors (Langeveld et al. 2004) found that 54 per cent worried about having a relapse, 43 per cent worried about the health of their future children and 50 per cent reported worries about having another cancer when they got older. Women worried more about cancer-specific concerns than men, a finding that was echoed by Hudson et al. (2003). In Langeveld et al.'s (2004) study, survivors and controls did not differ in their mean scores for general health concerns, but this masked some noteworthy findings at the level of individual items. Survivors were found to worry more than the comparison group about whether they were as healthy as their peers, their fertility, getting or changing a job, and obtaining life or medical insurance. Perhaps more surprisingly, survivors were found to worry less than the comparison group about some minor health complaints and about dying, how their body looked, their parents' health, and losing friends. This pattern of results is broadly consistent with several other studies in this area (Weigers et al. 1998; Zebrack and Chesler 2002). In Zebrack and Chesler's (2002) study, adolescent and young adult survivors of childhood cancer rated themselves high on happiness, feeling useful, life satisfaction and ability to cope as a result of having had cancer, though they expressed concerns about the impact of their illness on their family and fears about a second cancer. Survivors who had completed treatment a greater number of years ago seem to have fewer cancer specific worries than those who had completed treatment more recently, suggesting that these concerns become less prominent with the passage of time (Langeveld et al. 2004).

Conclusions

Research on late effects of childhood cancer has primarily taken two routes: one, an identification of the physical pathologies associated with having cancer and its treatment in childhood, and the second, focused on the psychosocial problems of people who survive cancer in childhood. It is important not to discount the psychosocial difficulties experienced by certain groups of survivors, and it is also important that research continues to improve our understanding of the factors that contribute to the risk of psychosocial difficulties so that appropriate resources may be directed to the support and care of those who experience them. However, such studies tell us relatively little about the issues that survivors find distressing, nor do they tell us much about the majority of survivors who do not experience pronounced or enduring difficulties. In considering the evidence on psychosocial outcomes for survivors of childhood cancer and their families, the picture that emerges suggests that adverse psychosocial outcomes are far from being an inevitable result of survivorship. Survivors are at elevated risk of some adverse psychosocial outcomes, but much of this risk is largely confined to certain sub-groups and only a minority of survivors will experience pronounced or enduring psychosocial difficulties. This is a remarkable finding and one that highlights the inadequacy of individual psychopathology as the sole model for investigating and understanding the experiences of survivors. It also points to the importance of treatment and diagnostic issues in understanding the pathways to poor psychosocial outcomes. This does not diminish the significance of adverse outcomes for the individuals who are affected, but it does highlight the importance of considering other ways of representing the experiences of survivors and their families. For example the psycho-oncology literature has promoted a deficit model of survivorship, but it is unclear whether survivors themselves approach their experiences from a deficit-centred perspective.

Promising lines of theorizing are offered by the literature on adults' experiences of chronic illness and on adults' experiences of cancer survivorship, including processes or ordering of meaning, identity, strategic management and biography. There is only a very small body of empirical evidence as yet to support this kind of work with children, but this does indicate that narrative-based research will be a vital complement to the kinds of survey-based work that has predominated thus far. What is clear is that childhood cancer does not 'stop' when it is deemed cured; the boundaries between wellness and sickness are, as Frank (1995) suggests, heavily blurred.

5 Families' experiences of childhood cancer

We noted in Chapter 1 that the new social studies of childhood fails to give adequate place to the experiences of families. We also argued that the experiences of families in relation to childhood cancer have been inappropriately theorized within psychology. In this chapter we suggest that the needs and roles of families of children with cancer have been inadequately conceptualized by traditional approaches to investigating the psychosocial aspects of childhood. Conducted mainly within discourses of psychopathology, traditional approaches have tended to characterize families' experiences of childhood cancer in terms of 'maladjustment' and 'coping', but have done little to illuminate the processes involved in how parents and siblings live with life-threatening childhood illness. In other areas, the research literature tends to treat parents solely as proxy sources of their children's views, and the complexity of their roles as caregivers and individuals in their own right has been ignored.

We attempt to recharacterize the families of children with cancer, drawing attention to how their roles, identities and social obligations position them in relation to the medical world, and highlight the emotional and other forms of work carried out by family members, including the protection of their own, and their ill child's, identity. Drawing on various bodies of empirical and theoretical work, including the literature on informal carers, we suggest ways of rethinking our understanding of the experiences of families.

Traditional approaches to the experiences of parents

Traditional approaches have attempted to estimate the proportion of parents likely to experience psychological difficulties while their child is on treatment and in the months after treatment has finished. These approaches explore the links between parental adjustment and individual characteristics, such as personality traits, coping styles, illness perceptions or familial cohesiveness (Grootenhuis and Last 1997; Kazak et al. 1998; Sloper 2000b). A similar vein of research has pursued associations between parental adjustment (particularly maternal adjustment) and child adjustment (Sawyer et al. 1998).

Studies prior to the 1980s tended to indicate that parents of children with cancer experienced considerable psychological distress. More recent evidence suggests that parents experience considerable distress in the immediate aftermath of their child's diagnosis (Fife 1987; Manne et al. 1995; Sloper 1996), but for most this is temporary. Though most studies suggest that the distress experienced by parents whose children are (temporarily) off treatment is generally lower, there may be a temporary increase in levels of anxiety among parents just around the time treatment ends (Grootenhuis and Last 1997). However, many investigations of parent psychosocial adjustment have been uncontrolled, small-scale studies with poorly selected samples. It is possible that estimates from such studies are unreliable, or underpowered to detect small but clinically important psychological difficulties. A recent exception is a population-based controlled study of 243 families of a child with cancer and 278 control families conducted in New Zealand (Dockerty et al. 2000). Parents of children with cancer reported their mental health as being significantly lower than control parents, but the magnitude of these differences was small (2.2 for mothers and 1.9 for fathers on the General Health Questionnaire, a scale which has a maximum possible score of 36). The authors conclude that as a whole, parents showed considerable resilience to mental health problems, but note that some sub-groups were not doing as well as others.

Studies that have aimed to identify risk factors for psychological distress suggest the following may place parents at elevated risk:

- parental employment problems (Sloper 2000b);
- lower levels of social support (Dockerty et al. 2000; Fife et al. 1987; Frank et al. 2001);
- child behaviour problems (Manne et al. 1995), low family cohesiveness (Manne et al. 1995; Sloper 2000b);
- time since diagnosis (Fife et al. 1987; Sawyer et al. 1997);
- increased perceptions of illness strain, perceived life threat; perceived treatment intensity (Kazak et al. 1998; Sloper 2000b; Taïeb et al. 2003);
- avoidant/passive thought or coping styles (Norberg et al. 2005).

Again, much work that aims to identify risk factors for distress has been of poor methodological quality. Most studies of parents have been too small to undertake rigorous sub-group analyses, for example, of different tumour types. In addition, caution is needed in interpreting causal pathways in studies that generate weak-to-moderate associations in variables such as distress and illness perceptions and distress and coping, as these are unlikely to be entirely separate constructs (Norberg et al. 2005).

Though not without its methodological shortcomings, this body of work has been important in drawing practitioners' attention to the distress that some parents experience during their child's illness. It has also been useful in identifying some of the factors that may help to predict those parents who are likely to experience difficulties, so that appropriate support might be made available (Kazak et al. 2003), but the danger of stigmatizing must be taken into account as this will add to the difficulties of such families.

In identifying psychopathology and individual deficits as the major feature of interest in families who experience catastrophic childhood illness, this work runs risk of pathologizing parents' experiences: one line of research, for example, has involved identifying constellations of psychological difficulties in parents, which, though too mild in themselves to be classified as clinically significant, are nevertheless considered sufficient to warrant further psychiatric surveillance (Kazak et al. 1998). Perhaps the most important weaknesses of this approach, however, are the very limited scope of inquiry, which tends to neglect the sociocultural context of caring for a child with chronic illness, and the use of methods that do little to access the meanings that parents themselves give to their experiences (Young et al. 2002).

Quality of life approaches

Quality of life approaches, with their focus on the measurement of subjective well-being across a number of life domains rather than a limited focus on psychopathology, offer the prospect of moving to a more appropriate way of representing the experience of parents. As discussed in Chapter 3, recent years have seen some much-needed progress in the development of measures to assess health-related quality of life (HRQoL) in children with cancer. There is, however, a continuing tendency to seek parents' views only as proxies for their children, and few instruments have so far been developed to assess how the quality of parents' own lives is affected by their children's illnesses. Many so-called parent quality-of-life scales are actually child quality-of-life instruments, while others assess only a limited range of the possible dimensions of quality of life (Streisand et al. 2001). Items have often been derived from instruments produced for other purposes and without the benefit of parents' narrative accounts of their experiences to inform instrument development. The initial selection of items for some measures has largely relied on health professionals' views of what is important to families (Wright 1993). Such practices risk producing instruments that fail to measure what is important to parents, and which overlook their unique status as carers, the complexities of their roles, and the particular difficulties they encounter in caring for a child with cancer.

Experiences of parents of children with cancer

While there is a clear need for rigorous qualitative research on parents' accounts of having a child with cancer, much of the existing qualitative literature is thus far disappointing in both quality and quantity. Some papers continue to draw heavily on the individualistic concepts of traditional approaches such as coping and adjustment, while others suffer from problems of poor study design, reporting or interpretation. However, a growing body of better quality work (some of which has investigated the experiences of parents of children with serious illnesses other than cancer), is now beginning to show how the roles and identities of parents position them in relation to the medical world, and how this impacts on their experience of having a child with cancer. This work underlines our argument that to exclude parents from the study of childhood is to provide only a partial account of experiences of childhood as a social category.

Being a carer, being a parent

For virtually all parents, becoming a parent of a child with cancer is a striking biographical transition. It requires a fundamental redefining of their self-identities (Van Dongen-Melman et al. 1998; Young et al. 2002) and represents the beginning of a 'passage through crisis' (Davis 1963). In our study of 20 mothers of children with cancer (Young et al. 2003), mothers contrasted the certainty and control of their pre-illness lives with their post-diagnosis lives. Their narratives emphasized how the diagnosis activated a process in constructing a new self-identity which brought with it new responsibilities and roles. The new self-identity was reflexively constructed, grounded in the experiential realities of childhood cancer, drawing on culturally prescribed expectations of carers and mothers, and modified through a 'cycle of reappraisals and revisions in the light of new information and knowledge' (Williams and Calnan 1996: 1617). Our analysis suggests that there are characteristic features of the self-identity and experiences of the mother of a child with cancer. Although they are not themselves ill, parents experience many of the consequences of chronic illness, including biographical disruption, compromise in role function and deterioration in quality of life. They are heavily involved in forms of work related to their child's illness, including emotional and care-giving work.

Having a child with cancer requires a parent to assume a complex range of overlapping and sometimes contradictory roles. One important role for parents is caring, involving obligations and responsibilities for the physical and emotional well-being of the ill child. These obligations are reflexively constructed, but also socially and culturally produced. (Young et al. 2002).

The literature on informal carers, (for example, Twigg and Atkin 1994), some of the earliest examples of which focused on the experiences of parents caring for disabled children (Voysey 1975), provides some useful conceptual tools for theorizing the experiences of parents. Studies in this vein have highlighted the cost, energy and skilfulness involved in providing care and the consequences for carers' own well-being (McKeever and Miller 2004). However, 'caring' also has some limitations as a theoretical construct – for example in emphasizing parents' caring role, it does not adequately recognize the extent to which, as we discussed in Chapter 4, children are not simply passive recipients of care, but are also active in the strategic management and emotional and biographical tasks of their illness. We propose that it is more appropriate to conceive of parents as participating in the strategic co-management of childhood cancer, as well as in wider forms of work related to the illness.

Strategic co-management of childhood cancer and the social construction of childhood cancer

Parents undertake or facilitate the strategic management (Bury 1982) of childhood cancer. In our study, parents reported managing the day-to-day routines and practical requirements of their child's treatment, including ensuring that their child: was properly fed; complied with treatment; did not become overly distressed; had access to supportive and competent medical and nursing care, and to education and friendships (Young et al. 2003). Much of the work arises from the obligations associated with the social construction of parenting, particularly the social construction of parenting in a crisis.

A key obligation generated by the diagnosis of childhood cancer is the need felt by parents to be physically close to the sick child at all times. In the weeks or months following the diagnosis, many mothers remain vigilantly at their children's sides around the clock (Faulkner et al. 1995). Some researchers have applied labels such as 'separation anxiety' to this phenomenon, implying that it is undesirable or even dysfunctional for parents to maintain a near constant presence at their children's sides (Patistea et al. 2000). However, we suggest that it is more appropriate to characterize this phenomenon as a socially generated and reflexively constructed obligation of 'proximity'. In explaining why they take on this role, mothers cite the special character of the mother–child relationship and the importance of their presence in comforting their child. It also serves as a demonstration of the adequacy of their parenting when there is little they can otherwise do to ensure their child's recovery (Young et al. 2002).

> And she's holding my hand day and night to say don't go away, don't leave me alone, and I couldn't leave her like that so I was there

with her until they allowed me to come home with her. And I was there for more than 2 months.
(Mother of female patient, aged 4, cited in Young et al. 2002: 1838)

Mothers of young people spoke of their own need to be there or keep watch over their child, even if their presence was not always desired; their own felt obligations overrode attempts by their children to limit their roles.

I can't leave her on her own, I can't. She tells me sometimes, 'Why don't you just go home?' And I can't. I just think, I couldn't leave a child in hospital, I just wouldn't, I couldn't sleep at home.
(Mother of female patient, aged 17, cited in Young et al. 2002: 1838)

Parents also experience an obligation to secure their child's cooperation with treatment, including getting them to take medicines and submit to unpleasant procedures (Young et al. 2002). They may have extreme difficulties in achieving this:

The only way I could get her to do it, and sometimes now I wish I didn't say it to her, but the only way I could actually get her ... and I sat down with her one day and I said 'You do know that unless you let the doctors give you your treatment to you you'll die' ... I wouldn't recommend anybody to do that but it worked ... I mean a child psychiatrist would probably say that was completely the wrong thing to do ... but I was just desperate and nobody else could give me any advice because I'd tried everything.
(Mother of female patient, aged 5, quoted in Young et al. 2002: 1839)

Socially positioned as the guardians of their child's 'futurity' (McKeever and Miller 2004), parents are acutely conscious of the potential consequences of being unable to manage their children's cooperation. These seem to go beyond the everyday scrutiny to which mothers are subject as their children's 'accountable agents' (Voysey 1975). This role is just one of the many social constructions of parenthood and childhood cancer that parents have to negotiate.

One of the key contributions that a critical, interpretive and reflexive approach to understanding childhood cancer can make is in revealing these social constructions of childhood cancer and their implications for people's experiences. As Bury (2001) explains, lay people's responses to illness frequently draw upon, and in turn constitute culturally available concepts of disease and illness that powerfully influence the fashioning of narratives. Images, mythologies and narratives about children abound in popular media, both reflecting and constructing contemporary ideals of childhood. These representations of childhood structure the cultural and moral climate of parenting (James et al. 1998), and shape the care-giving work of parents (Burman 1994).

Jenks (1996a) distinguishes two discourses of children that emerge from historical and cross-cultural analysis: Dionysian and Apollonian. Dionysian discourses portray children as 'little devils' – inherently unsocialized, naughty and unruly beings. Apollonian constructions, by contrast, represent children as 'little angels', who are born good, innocent and highly vulnerable. Media stories of childhood illness and disability typically invoke powerful Apollonian visions of children, and involve inspirational narratives of children heroically overcoming obstacles. Romanticized images of the family life of children with a serious illness, with parents positioned as endlessly self-sacrificing, children as invariably optimistic and brave, can involve serious distortions (Moller 1996). Rolland (1997) has argued that these idealized portrayals of successful coping strategies represent adult fantasies that may be experienced as oppressive by children and families who find themselves unable to cope in this way.

In the newspaper accounts of childhood cancer studied in Dixon-Woods et al.'s (2003) study, certain representations become privileged while others were suppressed: it becomes unseemly, for example, to report a child with cancer as being anything other than 'brave' and uncomplaining; to do otherwise would involve violating the dominant cultural metaphor of stoicism. Cancer itself is represented as an assault on the entitlements and category-bound activities of childhood, with parents, community, and doctors enlisted as confederates in the battle against this evil. Little conflict between the confederates is reported, supporting a dominant metaphor of unity in the face of threat to innocence.

Media accounts thus allow insight into the socially constructed nature of the idealized image of childhood and into the prescribed norms of managing response to threats to childhood. This response involves the marginalization of parents into the role of a resource in the battle against cancer; little attention is given to their own needs. Popular images of childhood cancer and parenthood promoted by media accounts may be a source of tension for parents, sometimes creating public expectations and stereotypes that are difficult to fulfil. For these reasons, parents may find it difficult to give voice to their own needs or aspects of their own experiences (Dixon-Woods et al. 2003). Indeed, one of the obligations of parenting a child with cancer is to be selfless and devoted; in common with parenting a child with disabilities, parents (and particularly women) are expected to forfeit or modify paid employment and devote themselves entirely to their caring role (McKeever and Miller 2004).

Children's experiences and parents' experiences are thus intimately intertwined. This is especially evident in the emotional work that parents undertake, where there is strong evidence of emotional interdependence, with parents' own emotional well-being tied to that of their child. An important obligation created by this is the need to keep children entertained, in the belief that this is vital to promoting psychological health (Young et al. 2002). Our study (Young et al. 2002) also identified that parents perceive an obligation to manage their own identity as hopeful, optimistic and strong. This included presenting a 'cheerful' disposition. Helping children to 'pass as normal', as we identified in Chapter 4, was another important obligation. Work thus far suggests that parents tend to take on a role akin to that of 'alert assistant', working in subtle or invisible ways to protect their child's identity, or to represent their status as 'ordinary' (Williams 2000; Young et al. 2002).

The parental performance of obligations is crucially influenced by the social conditions of medical treatment for childhood cancer. Parents may find it difficult to challenge medical authority or violate other boundaries of the clinical world, and may find themselves cast in an intensely conflicted role as their children's advocates, where their dependence on professionals means that they must accept that they are subordinates, but on the other hand are expected to 'speak up' for their child. In our study (Young et al. 2002), a mother from a South Asian background described how she felt unable to insist that nurses attend to her child's needs immediately, even when these were pressing.

> I was really very upset about it because I wanted to do the best for her and yet I couldn't because I just didn't have the assertiveness to say look my daughter wants this now, could she have it? I couldn't do that.
>
> (Mother quoted in Young et al. 2002: 1839)

McKeever and Miller (2004) provide an interesting Bourdieusian analysis of this phenomenon, arguing that parents acquire a feel for the medical game and suppress displays of anger or criticism that would be expected of mothers in other fields. The potency of the medical agenda is, therefore, subscribed to by all parties. Investment in their children's survival means that parents accommodate to the demands of the treatment in a reflexive process that weighs its pros and cons, but perhaps more importantly involves an reordering of meaning that transforms the very basis of their judgements. It is not simply that all other concerns are subordinate to their child's survival; in accommodating to their children's treatment, parents are engaging in something that needs to be understood in the language of belief, trust and faith, and it is these concepts that underpin their relationship with medicine and its practitioners.

Biographical work and the search for meaning

A characteristic task undertaken by parents of children with cancer is the reordering of meaning in the face of hugely threatening disruption. Current evidence suggests that parents perform biographical work not only for themselves but also in support of their ill children. Based on their long-itudinal work on parents' responses to childhood cancer, Martinson and Cohen (1988) suggest that the everyday parental concern with protecting their child's physical and emotional well-being helps to normalize the parenting role, and serves to rekindle a sense of familiarity in the face of the disruption caused by the illness (Martinson and Cohen 1988). Families of ill children may also experience 'grief' for their previous lives in which former aspirations could be fulfilled (Van Dongen-Melman et al. 1998), in the same way as people with chronic illness grieve for their former selves (Kelly 1986).

> . . . because it's like a grief you go through at first. It's a grief for a former life where you were sort of carefree, you had four healthy children, everything was pretty much progressing as you hoped and one day everything changes and you feel like losing a child.
> (Mother of 9-year-old boy, quoted in Dixon-Woods et al. 2003: 157)

Parents also engage in narrative work to try to address questions of 'why me?' and 'why now?' (Pill and Stott 1982; Tuckett 1976). Williams's (1984) classic paper on narrative reconstructions undertaken by people with chronic illness showed how people's narratives tend to reorder events so that they tell a potentially plausible and coherent story of why the disease happened to them. This type of biographical work is a key feature of childhood cancer. Comaroff and Maguire (1981) showed how parents identified environmental causes for their child's cancer, and other work has suggested that some parents also wonder if they themselves are to blame for failing to protect their child from hazards during pregnancy and early childhood (Dixon-Woods et al. 2001). Yeh (2003), in an interview study of 32 Taiwanese parents, found that some parents blamed themselves, attributing the cancer their own negligence in caring, genetic heritage, or unhealthy lifestyle. Religious belief contributed to some parents believing that their child's illness was a punishment for their past sin. In this way, the diagnosis can threaten the biographies of both parents and children.

Gendering of parenting

Childhood illness appears to amplify traditional gender divisions of labour as mothers (particularly) relinquish other roles to take on most of the caregiving tasks associated with the illness (Brown and Barbarin 1996). Feminist theorizing on the family and motherhood has identified how for women in particular, motherhood is both a regulator of their lives and a major component of their self-identity (Richardson 1993). Though women with children increasingly adopt roles outside the domestic sphere, mothers' emotional identification with their children remains strong, and notions of maternal self-sacrifice in 'putting the children first' and of children's 'best interests' (Sclater et al. 1999) remain powerful in both public and private discourses about motherhood and childhood, as we identified earlier. Williams (2002) shows how gender is implicated in the family's response to illness and everyone 'just accepts' that mothers will be in charge of helping children to deal with their disease. However, mothers often experience significant role strain in fulfilling their obligations to their sick child: they are unable to perform basic caring tasks for their other children and many experience guilt and regret about this (Faulkner et al. 1995; Sloper 1996; Yeh et al. 2000).

Although research on fathers is notably lacking, a very small body of research is beginning to emerge. Jones and Neil-Urban's (2003) small focus-group study of fathers demonstrates that fathers' narratives are very similar in form to those obtained in studies conducted mainly with mothers, covering issues such as the diagnosis, the impact of the cancer on the family, and so on. Interestingly, in this study, fathers described taking on much more aggressive advocacy roles and emphasized the need to 'stand up' to medical personnel, suggesting that the acceptance of the subordinate and compliant role we described earlier might be gendered.

> I have gone head to head with many doctors in the last year and a half. I've said if I can keep my daughter from being stuck one more time, then you're going to have to explain to me why you have to do this or why you can't give her this injection while she's out for some other procedure.
>
> (Father quoted in Jones and Neil-Urban 2003: 52)

It is clear that fathers too have to negotiate expectations that are ambiguous or conflicting, particularly in reconciling their perceived obligations as a breadwinner with their own felt need to be with their sick child, and to care for their other children (Chesler and Parry 2001; Jones and Neil-Urban 2003). These studies also confirm the strain on marriage and relationships identified in work with mothers, but Jones and Neil-Urban's study described the difficulties men may have in giving voice to their emotions and, in a striking parallel to parents concealing their emotions from children, fathers described concealing their emotions from their partners in order to appear strong and reliable.

Research on fathers of ill children suggests that social-cultural aspects of the healthcare system shape or reinforce gendered patterns of care-giving.

Health professionals may lack experience in dealing with fathers, with the result that they are often left out of the communication chain and receive much of their information second hand (Chesler and Parry 2001; Faulkner et al. 1995). These difficulties may be exacerbated by their non-domestic obligations, or when the father no longer resides in the family home.

In a detailed and insightful study of the gendered patterns in which mothers and fathers deal with their emotions after the diagnosis of their child's cancer, Reay et al. (1998) note how these gendered role expectations, coupled with individual inclinations, shaped mothers' and fathers' emotional lives after the diagnosis. Fathers' and mothers' accounts exhibited a range of emotional responses but there were important commonalities in the way that men as a group, and women as a group, dealt with childhood cancer. Though fathers described experiencing intense and difficult feelings, many tended to avoid expressing them, distancing themselves emotionally from the illness. Accounts of mothers and fathers focused on father's reluctance to talk about the illness (perhaps reflecting the 'need to be strong' described earlier). In some cases fathers minimized the significance of the diagnosis, while mothers tended to become highly emotionally engaged with their child and everyday aspects of their life and treatment. This could sometimes result in a degree of friction, incomprehension and estrangement between couples.

Services

A body of work has highlighted how the adequacy of healthcare service provision can play a key role in mediating the experiences of parents of children with cancer. This includes the quality of play and educational services for children, informational and community support, and organizational aspects of services, such as reduced delays in treatment and improvements to the 'hotel' aspects of services (Dixon-Woods et al. 2001; Enskar et al. 1997c). Qualitative research is also beginning to show how the everyday social and organizational aspects of health services can either undermine or support parents, and how good quality services, including parent–professional relationships, are essential in supporting the functioning of parents in their caring role.

Work with parents caring for children who had been admitted to hospital for surgery has shown how parents sometimes engage in personally costly strategies to ensure cooperation and avoid conflict during the hospitalization of their child (Atkin and Ahmad 2000; Callery 1997). The poor quality of some of the 'hotel' aspects of hospital services can undermine their attempts at normalization. For example, poor quality hospital food can result in parental anxiety about the adequacy of the child's diet for their recovery. Staff who are skilled in establishing successful relationships with children play a crucial role in gaining their cooperation with unpleasant procedures, thereby helping to relieve parents of the burden of enlisting their reluctant child's cooperation (Young et al. 2002).

There is some evidence pointing to the financial strains associated with caring for a child with cancer. In an Australian study, Cohn et al. (2003) found that families bore increased travel, food, accommodation and communication costs and faced a loss of income as a result of one or both parents having to give up their job or take time off work. A similar study of families in New Zealand found that the average extra expenditure amounted to 13 per cent of family income (Dockerty et al. 2003).

Parents' experiences of 'late effects'

Investigations of the psychosocial late effects of childhood cancer on parents have mostly focused on rates of depression, anxiety, coping, family functioning, post-traumatic stress disorder and parents' worries and concerns. Studies of late effects for parents have been considerably fewer than those of children and most have typically involved samples of 100 families or fewer.

For most psychological domains there is little or no convincing evidence of lasting psychological difficulties among parents of survivors (Kupst et al. 1995; Sawyer et al. 1997, 1998, 2000). Grootenhuis and Last (1997) identified seven studies which had examined depression, anxiety, coping and family functioning in parents of survivors. None of these found evidence of poor psychosocial outcomes in parents of survivors compared to parents of controls or population norms. However, these studies have used small samples and may, therefore, be underpowered to detect small but possibly clinically important psychological difficulties in parents. In addition, these studies do not allow for sub-group analyses of the form that have been important in identifying survivors at elevated risk of psychosocial difficulties.

By contrast, several studies have suggested that parents of survivors may have elevated rates of post-traumatic stress disorder (PTSD) compared with controls and population norms, and may be more likely to experience PTSD than their surviving children (Barakat et al. 1997; Kazak et al. 1997; Taïeb et al. 2003). Factors most strongly associated with risk of PTSD include parents' beliefs about the threat that the illness posed and continues to pose to their child's life, the perceived intensity of the treatment, family income and social support available to the family (Goldenberg Libov et al. 2002; Taïeb et al. 2003). It should be noted however, that the credibility and specificity of the diagnosis of PTSD has been contested, and though officially classified as a mental disorder, clinicians and researchers are far from agreement about the value of PTSD as a diagnostic category (Summerfield 2001).

The finding that beliefs about the illness may have a particularly important role in the risk of PTSD for parents is broadly consistent with qualitative and quantitative evidence that suggests some parents of survivors may experience enduring concerns and worries about the illness. For parents in Dixon-Woods et al.'s (2003) study, the threat to the future that cancer represented was a very powerful one. Long-term effects of the child's illness and treatment become potent symbols of their altered status, and these, coupled with ever-present fears of disease recurrence continue to taint the biographies of parents and children (Faulkner et al. 1995; Martinson and Cohen 1988; Van Dongen-Melman et al. 1998).

Van Dongen-Melman et al. (1998), in a qualitative study, found that parents of survivors experienced a sense of loss for their former lives and for their child's former self. The experience of the illness was found to have eliminated parents' sense of invulnerability about their own lives and that of their family, and for some there were continuing fears that the illness might return. The authors highlight the fluid and context-dependent ways in which several parents dealt with their situation and suggest that families may derive benefit from using a range of strategies at different times, including both avoidance and confrontation of the illness. They note that dispositional measures of coping may be inadequate for capturing the complexity and fluidity of parents' strategies. While this study points to the difficulties that become a feature of parents' lives, Van Dongen-Melman et al. (1998) note that parents' accounts were not exclusively defined by uncertainty and worries about their child. Indeed, several parents attested to their child's strength and to how the experience of parenting a child with cancer had provided the impetus to revaluate their lives and priorities, and brought a greater closeness in the relationships of some parents

Summarizing the evidence in this area, Grootenhuis and Last (1997) point to parents' fears about possible relapse and infertility in their child, and feelings of loneliness and uncertainty about the future. Uncertainty was also prominent in a recent study by Zebrack et al. (2002b). This mixed qualitative and quantitative study found that like most parents, mothers of survivors worried about their children's physical and psychosocial well-being. But these worries were shaped and intensified by issues that are of particular concern to survivors and their families, including relapse, the possibility of a second cancer, infertility, difficulties in gaining health insurance and possible psychosocial difficulties experienced by their child. Analyses of the quantitative data suggested that mothers' worries were most strongly associated, not with the physical consequences of their child's illness, but with their perceptions of their child's worries about the illness, and the meanings mothers attached to their own and their child's experience of the illness. Ressler et al. (2003) reported that many parents continued to be concerned about their child's health and the risk of cancer recurrence, and valued the opportunity to continue to attend health appointments with their adult children who had survived cancer.

Traditional approaches to the experiences of siblings

It is commonly claimed that siblings of children with cancer have been overlooked or neglected by researchers. This claim no longer stands up to scrutiny, as there is now a large number of studies of well siblings, some dating back to the 1960s, investigating associations between growing up in a family affected by chronic childhood illness and adverse psychological outcomes (for example, Wold and Townes 1969). However, much work continues to be dominated by a quest to find evidence of psychopathology, and, with a few notable exceptions, siblings' experiences of growing up in families affected by chronic childhood illness and what forms of support are likely to be helpful to them have been little researched.

Several studies have reported an increased risk of psychopathology and adjustment problems for siblings of chronically ill children (Cohen et al. 1994; Fife et al. 1987; Houtzager et al. 2003; Spinetta 1981). However, other studies have found no evidence to conclude that siblings are at increased risk of psychosocial difficulties (Dolgin et al. 1997; Horowitz and Kazak 1990), and a few studies have suggested that some aspects of siblings' social functioning may be enhanced by the experience of having a brother or sister with a life-threatening illness (Harder and Bowditch 1982; Kramer 1984). Houtzager et al. (1999) and Sharpe and Rossiter (2002) point to the methodological problems that have beset research in this area, including the use of short-term follow-ups, inappropriate study designs, sampling problems and inconsistencies in how key outcomes have been operationalized.

Several reviews of the evidence have been conducted to attempt to interpret this contradictory evidence (Houtzager et al. 1999; Sharpe and Rossiter 2002; Williams 1997). A meta-analysis of 51 studies (Sharpe and Rossiter 2002) deserves special attention. Healthy siblings of children with chronic illness were found to be at slightly increased risk of adverse outcomes (depression and anxiety, reduced peer activities and developmental delay) compared with controls and with normative data, but there was a great deal of variation between studies in estimates of the degree of risk encountered by siblings, and parent reports tended to produce higher risk estimates than child self-reports. In suggesting that the difficulties encountered by siblings are unlikely to put them at risk of severe psychopathology, this meta-analysis further highlights the limitations of understanding the lives of siblings largely in terms of psychopathology (Houtzager et al. 1999; Sloper and While 1996). Nevertheless, it is important that professionals and parents remain alert to the possible emotional distress and other difficulties that some siblings of children with chronic illness may experience.

Another strand of work has attempted to identify factors that may place siblings at elevated risk of emotional and psychosocial difficulties. Evidence suggests that the greater an ill child's care and support needs, the greater the risk to sibling functioning (Sharpe and Rossiter 2002; Sloper and While 1996). A review of the evidence (Williams 1997) suggests that poor sibling adjustment is associated with maternal depression, poor family cohesion, high levels of family stress and younger age of siblings. However, an interesting study by the same author found that of the wide range of variables examined (family socio-economic status, family cohesion, and sibling age, mood, illness knowledge and attitudes, self-esteem and social support), family socio-economic status and family cohesion were most strongly associated with parent-reported sibling behaviour problems (Williams et al. 2002). Family socio-economic status was a particularly important influence on sibling behaviour problems: through its moderating effect on maternal mood, it was found to have indirect effects on family cohesion, which was the second most important risk factor for sibling behaviour problems.

The authors sound a note of caution about psychosocial interventions to improve sibling adjustment, suggesting that interventions which do not take into account the multiple stresses faced by families on low incomes are unlikely to have much success. It should be noted that Williams et al.'s (2002) study was based in the USA where health and social welfare provision for low income families compares unfavourably with the UK and western Europe. Nevertheless, a study on risk factors for sibling maladjustment conducted in the UK also found that the lack of resources typically experienced by low-income families, such as lack of access to a car for travelling to hospital visits, was an important risk factor for sibling adjustment difficulties (Sloper and While 1996).

Experiences of siblings

Little research has investigated the quality of life of siblings. However, several qualitative studies have investigated the experience of having a brother or sister with cancer. Much of this work points to the disrupting effect of the illness on siblings' lives and concepts of loss and change in roles and relationships are particularly prominent in these studies.

Loss and separation

Siblings in Faulkner et al.'s (1995) study described how they missed their parents' presence during acute phases of the illness when parents usually spent as much time as possible in hospital at the bedside of the sick child. Keenly aware of the strain their parents were under, siblings did not wish to add to parents' difficulties by exhibiting signs of their own distress and several commented that they lacked anyone with whom they could share their worries and concerns. Kramer (1984) also notes that siblings in her study described feelings of anxiety, loneliness, confusion and sadness as a consequence of their separation from their parents.

Sloper's (2000a) unusually large qualitative study of 94 well siblings highlighted the considerable disruption they experienced in their day-to-day routines. Their accounts pointed to restrictions in their opportunities to socialize with friends, and missing the companionship of their ill brother or sister. As with Faulkner's study, one of the most prominent aspects of Sloper's findings was siblings' accounts of lessening attention from parents as their energies became directed towards ensuring the well-being of their ill child (Faulkner et al. 1995; Sloper 2000a). Many siblings experienced a range of conflicting emotions as a result, including resentment and anger, but not all siblings were overly perturbed about the decline in parental attention, and some took pains to demonstrate that they understood why their parents' attention was focused elsewhere. Younger children in particular may be more prone to overt displays of jealousy.

> J. used to get very jealous 'Why is [child] getting more attention than what I am, why is he getting more toys and presents?' because a lot of people used to come and visit and bring presents and cards. 'Why is he getting all that and why am I not getting anything?'
> (Mother of boy, aged 5, quoted in Dixon-Woods et al. 2003: 158)

For others, the loss of parental attention was coupled with decline in their feelings of certainty and security, and an increased sense of their own and their family's vulnerability. There were no straightforward answers to siblings' questions about the causes of their brother's or sister's illness and a few worried that they themselves might also contract cancer. More commonly, siblings feared that their brother or sister might die as a result of the illness, and 18 months after the diagnosis several continued to express considerable concerns about the possibility of relapse or death. Similar fears of illness and death were found by Koch-Hattem (1986) in her study of well siblings of children with cancer.

> I used to think I had all kinds of things . . . I used to sit and think, 'Oh no, what if I have . . .' I really thought I had something. I was afraid to tell anybody' cause they'd think I was silly. But it was very real to me for a while.
> (Koch-Hattem 1986: 114)

Different tensions may arise at later stages of the illness when the ill child starts to recover, and when parents and siblings begin to direct their attention to rekindling a sense of normality and to minimizing the intrusion of illness in their lives. Inappropriate attention and support for siblings at this time may risk bringing the illness to centre stage again, and weaken their chances of re-establishing their role within the family and reclaiming the attention of their parents (Bluebond-Langner 1996). Bluebond-Langner (1996) suggests that in addition to identifying the support needs of siblings, it is important to realize that some of the difficulties they encounter may be inevitable.

> Much of what the well sibling feels in the way of lack of attention, disruption of family lifestyle, concern for the ill child, and fear of the illness's consequences may be not only unavoidable, but also appropriate.
>
> (Bluebond-Langner 1996: 266)

Resources, roles and relationships

An important theme running through accounts of well siblings concerns how relationships with parents and other family members are transformed by having a brother or sister with chronic illness (Bluebond-Langner 1996; Faulkner et al. 1995; Kramer 1984; Sloper 2000a). Sloper (2000a) has highlighted how siblings feel they have lost their normal childhood entitlements, including those to attention, that their needs are dismissed and that parents are irritable with them. This is underscored by the constant enquiries from friends and acquaintances about their brother's or sister's well being.

> They don't say, 'Hi, Sally, how are you?' It's 'Is your brother all right?' Sometimes it annoys me because they only know me because my brother is ill, not for things I've done or anything. I just have to walk through the door and it's 'Is your brother all right, how is he?'
>
> (Older sister, aged 14, Sloper 2000a: 301)

Kramer (1984) uses the concept of 'emotional realignment' to represent the transformed family relationships following the diagnosis, and prominent in the accounts of the well siblings she studied was an increase in their parents' expectations of them, particularly that they should tolerate the indulgences and allowances received by their brother or sister because of the illness.

Based on her ethnographic study of families of children with cystic fibrosis, Bluebond-Langner (1996) suggests that it is possible to gain insight into siblings' feelings about their changed status within the family, including their rights and responsibilities, by exploring how they handle concerns about the allocation of resources such as parental attention. She charts how the position of siblings changes with the ebbs and flows of the illness. During illness exacerbations, siblings inevitably fall outside the scope of their parents' attention. Some sense that their entitlements to parental attention are diminished by the illness, but, nonetheless, struggle with their desires for attention and parity with their sibling. For others the illness may fuel attempts to win back some attention by 'playing up', or through their own displays of 'illness'. Their diminished entitlements to parental attention and to reciprocity with their ill sibling means their role as sons or daughters, and as brothers or sisters, is kept in abeyance. As neither carers nor patients, well siblings may experience difficulties in finding an alternative role within the family.

According to Bluebond-Langner (1996) well siblings can only re-establish a claim to a share in their parents' attention, and to the other rights and privileges of childhood, if and when the acute phase of the illness begins to recede. At this time, well siblings join with their parents in working to normalize the illness by compartmentalizing its visible signs, by emphasizing the ways that the ill child is like other children and by avoiding talk about the illness. This can have important implications for their information and communication needs.

Information and communication

Information-giving encounters provide an opportunity for siblings to express any worries they may have, and to obtain reassurance (Sloper 2000a). However, there may be considerable difficulties in meeting the information and communication needs of siblings. In a small-scale survey of siblings of children with brain tumours, Freeman et al. (2000) found that one-third of siblings reported important problems with ways information have been given to them at the time of their brother's or sister's diagnosis. Other concerns for siblings included lack of information about their brother or sister's prognosis, appearance, moods, special needs at school and activity restrictions.

While survey work is invaluable in identifying common concerns among siblings, it does not, of course, give access to well siblings' narratives. Surveys are of limited value in exploring the process of communication from the perspective of siblings and they do not usually allow researchers to identify issues that they have not previously anticipated as being important. Few qualitative studies have explored in detail information needs and communication difficulties encountered by siblings of children with cancer. However Bluebond-Langner's (1996) work on the siblings of children with cystic fibrosis provides some valuable insights into the possible difficulties facing siblings of children with cancer.

Her work suggests that timing is crucial when broaching sensitive issues and that well siblings may experience difficulties in finding timely opportunities for discussion of 'life and death' questions. Around the time of diagnosis, or during acute phases of the illness, the focus of parents is very much on the ill child and siblings' information needs tend to be overlooked. Other studies lend support to this conclusion. When well siblings were asked to write about their psychosocial support needs they expressed a desire for more information about their brother's or sister's illness, and to be included in discussions about the illness and treatment (Murray 2002). Two-thirds of the siblings in another qualitative study said they would have liked more information in the days following a diagnosis of cancer (Sloper 2000a). However, it is important to note that the desire for more information may not be shared by all siblings; indeed, all of the children in Martinson et al.'s (1990) study who had a sibling recovering from cancer said they wanted no further information about the condition. The authors note that common factor in well siblings' accounts of information exchanges was the lack of power and feelings of exclusion they experienced, particularly their uncertainty about how to raise questions about their brother or sister's illness or what to say in response to questions from their friends.

There may also be considerable barriers to meeting well siblings' information and communication needs beyond the acute phase of the illness. Bluebond-Langner (1996) found that well siblings have questions about fundamental issues concerning the prognosis and progression of the illness, but in the recovery phase of the illness discussion of these is largely avoided because to raise them would undermine and threaten parents' and siblings' work to return their lives to normality.

Services and support for siblings

Several studies suggest that one of the most prominent priorities for well siblings is for a close and confiding relationship with someone with whom they can discuss their feelings when necessary, without the fear of burdening that person (Murray 2002; Sloper 2000a). However, Bluebond-Langner (1996) sounds a note of caution about approaches which uncritically advocate the pursuit of 'open communication', and about allowing concerns about age and stage of development to dominate decisions about what form of support to provide for siblings. She urges that support be based on the particular needs and experiences of siblings. Current evidence suggests that it is also important for siblings to have a focus outside the illness, to develop a role or position through which they can maintain their self-esteem and self-worth, or simply to have some respite from worries about their brother or sister's illness (Bluebond-Langner 1996; Sloper 2000a). This may be difficult to achieve because of the disrupting effects of the illness, but practical support to enable them to meet with friends or pursue everyday interests and activities may make a considerable contribution to promoting their well-being. A trial of an information and psychosocial support intervention for siblings of children with a chronic illness or disability has shown promising results in addressing their information and communication needs (Williams et al. 2003). A smaller-scale intervention by Barrera et al. (2002) has also shown promising results.

Conclusions

Traditional approaches to investigating families of children with cancer have been useful in highlighting the distress that family members may potentially experience. However, for research to move forward it is important to go beyond the limitations imposed by these dominant approaches. Shaped by a discourse of psychopathology and individualistic concepts, these approaches assess only a limited number of the many dimensions of families' experiences. They take little account of the priorities of parent and well siblings, and render uninteresting the remarkable situation of most who do not suffer lasting difficulties. In offering mainly individualized explanations of their distress, these approaches inevitably identify the source of families' difficulties as lying within themselves, and neglect the sociocultural factors that may have a major impact on the experience of living in a family of a child with cancer. For family members who are identified as maladjusted, their experience is represented as pathological or deviant, and they are constructed as suitable objects for clinical and moral surveillance.

Recognizing the social processes and the social context in which being a parent of a child with cancer takes place can contribute much to our understanding of their experiences. The literature on parents using qualitative methodologies that might assist with this project has been much better conducted and theorized than the research on children that we reported in Chapter 4, possibly reflecting the greater ease with which coherent narratives can be obtained from parents. The narratives of parents suggest that attention to the role and identity of parents, and how having a child with cancer threatens this role, may be particularly important. Even if a child makes a good recovery, his or her parents will remain the parents of a cancer 'survivor', learning to live with their altered self-identity, and with the realization that they could not fulfil the fundamental parental obligation of protection. As they search for the causes of their child's illness and reflect on the possibility of their own culpability (however unlikely), some have difficulty in reasserting their adequacy as parents. Incorporating the perspectives of parents into how we conceptualize and investigate their situation alerts us to the need to support them in ways that enable them to fulfil their roles and to regain their identities as 'adequate' parents. It also points to the part that the everyday organizational and social aspects of health services can play in this process.

Little of the work on well siblings acknowledges the tensions for parents and professionals in attending to the needs of both the ill child and their siblings. Writings frequently exhort professionals to remind parents about the needs of their well children, but during acute phases of the illness parents may be so overwhelmed with caring for their sick child and in dealing with their own emotions that they have little time or energy for their well children. In the context of life-threatening childhood illness such reminders may be asking the impossible, and unless sensitively handled and appropriately timed, may do much to undermine parents.

6   Communication in childhood cancer

Recent improvements in survival mean that the context of communicating about childhood cancer has transformed over the last few decades. Now, though cure is not guaranteed, children's chances of survival have improved dramatically and in many cases, questions about how to communicate are most appropriately considered in the context of how best to support children growing up with a chronic illness. Along with this, the increasingly demanding and arduous nature of treatments brings concerns about how best to prepare children for difficult and highly unpleasant treatments, some of which may last for several years.

In this chapter we will highlight several prominent features of the literature on communication with families in the context of childhood cancer, and discuss their implications. The literature on communicating with children is mostly under-theorized. Communication is treated in many studies and reviews as being largely synonymous with information-giving, or the transmission of 'facts' about the illness (Dixon-Woods 2001). Attempts are made to quantify and categorize the amount of information transmitted to children in an effort to gauge the 'openness of communication'. These approaches portray a particular view of communication and the parties involved that does not adequately capture the complexities of communication with young patients; very little attention is given to communication as a process of meaning construction, the perspectives the various parties bring to their encounters and how children, parents and health professionals interact and negotiate to build understandings that are meaningful to them.

The literature fails to problematize how the social positioning of children might affect this process and how children's access to communication is subject to challenges because of beliefs about their vulnerability, incompetence, and their status as dependants (James et al. 1998). At the same time children are active and agentic in the creation of meaning, and do not necessarily wait passively for information to be 'given' to them. We argue that accounts of communication are needed which represent communication as a process of meaning construction, and which scrutinize the roles and relationships of the various parties involved, the resources they draw upon and the sociocultural context in which communication takes place.

Giving children information

Many studies of 'communication' in childhood cancer have focused specifically on issues of information – how much children are given, how much they understand or retain, and the impact of information on their well-being. The literature is broadly grouped around three themes: disclosure of information about diagnosis and prognosis; information about late effects, and informational interventions to prepare children for medical procedures.

Patterns of disclosure of diagnosis and prognosis

'Telling versus not telling' debates have dominated approaches to communicating with children with cancer. Prior to the 1960s, it was often recommended that parents and professionals take a guarded approach to communicating with children: children were to be spared details of their illness and prognosis in an attempt to protect them from distress (Toch 1964). Recent years have seen a strong challenge to the view that children do not possess the competence to understand or remember details of their illness (Bird and Podmore 1990; Burman 1994; Carey 1985; Ornstein et al. 1997). This, together with debates about the rights and status of children (reviewed in detail in Chapter 7) have added impetus to approaches that advocate open communication, and we are now seeing approaches that strongly urge open information-giving (Alderson 1993b; BMA 2001) and greater inclusion of children in consultations.

How far these approaches are adopted in practice is perhaps uncertain, but some trends in information-giving are discernible in studies over time. Comaroff and Maguire (1981) found that the implications of the illness had been discussed with children in only six of the 60 families they studied. In a slightly later study, Chesler et al. (1986) found that over a third (36 per cent) of parents were considered to have engaged in 'relatively full disclosure of the illness'. Parents of older children reported giving more detailed information. Claflin and Barbarin (1991) found that in their study over half the children reported having been told nothing specific about their prognosis; 40 per cent reported being told about their illness (cancer or leukaemia) at diagnosis, with younger children considerably less likely to be told about their diagnosis.

A recent study in the UK (Clarke et al., in press) of 55 mothers of children newly diagnosed with acute lymphoblastic leukaemia distinguished four different styles of communication with children: full explanation including death (3 parents), most likely to be given to older children; providing factual information about cancer, without mentioning that the disease was serious or life-threatening (15 parents); providing ambiguous information (for example, telling children they had leukaemia but not mentioning that it was cancer)

(8 parents); and providing minimal information (for example, describing the illness as 'poorly blood') (17 parents). To what extent these styles persist over time or are initial ways of handling issues of disclosure is unclear. This study also provided little insight into why parents choose to adopt these communication styles.

A Dutch study published during the mid-1990s (Last and van Veldhuizen 1996) also provided evidence of the tendency for parents of younger children to report giving less detailed information. For example, use of the term 'cancer' tended to be avoided by parents of one-third of children aged 8–12 compared with one-fifth of parents of children aged 13–16. However, around 80 per cent of parents reported that their child had been given information about their prognosis, including the risk of relapse or recurrence, and the possibility that they might not recover. This figure was confirmed by the children's responses to the questionnaire, which indicated that across the whole sample about 80 per cent of children reported being informed that they might not get better, though younger children were still slightly less likely to be informed about details of their prognosis than older children. The authors note that parents felt it was important to give information to children in order to preserve their trust, to promote their child's acceptance of the illness, and because they felt their child had a right to be informed, while the most frequent reason for withholding information was a sense among parents that their child was too young to hear such frightening information.

Such concerns about developmental issues and children's vulnerability occupy a prominent place in writings about communicating with children (Rushforth 1999; Siegal and Peterson 1999) reflecting the tension between recognizing children's rights and protecting their well-being, which we discuss in more detail in Chapter 7. However, the empirical work in this area is limited. Most of the early studies focused on children with terminal illness who had been given very little or no information about their illness (Bluebond-Langner 1974; Spinetta 1974). These suggest that the extreme situation of total non-disclosure is associated with increased anxiety and isolation in children. Such studies have been of great importance in improving the psychosocial care of terminally ill children. However, with dramatically improved survival rates, these studies are perhaps less useful in answering more subtle questions about how to conduct communication in a way that is meaningful to children, and how to convey positive messages without being falsely reassuring or overly guarded.

Recent studies also leave many of these questions unanswered and have continued to focus on outcomes such as anxiety and knowledge, rather than how children give meaning to their illness and what resources they use in this process. In their study of information-giving, Last and van Veldhuizen (1996) found a series of low-to-moderate correlations between information-giving and psychosocial outcomes, suggesting that children who had been informed around the time of diagnosis that their illness was cancer, and had been given frank information about their prognosis, were less anxious and depressed than children who did not receive such information. Claflin and Barbarin (1991) found that levels of illness-related distress were broadly similar in all the age groups they studied, though children under 9 years were told considerably less about their illness and its treatment than older children. The authors conclude that this indicates that non-disclosure fails to ease the distress of younger children. However, this does exclude the possibility that the well-being of younger children could be adversely affected by giving them detailed information about their illness.

On the basis of their findings, Last and van Veldhuizen (1996) conclude that parents should be advised to discuss the diagnosis and prognosis openly with their child and should do so soon after the diagnosis has been confirmed. They recommend that parents use the word 'cancer' when talking about the illness and discuss with their children the possibility of dying from the disease, and point to the risk of accidental disclosures and the possible damaging consequences if children discover their diagnosis and prognosis from people other than parents or health professionals.

Information about late effects

Survey evidence from the USA suggests that adult survivors of childhood cancer are not well informed about basic aspects of their diagnosis and treatment (Kadan-Lottick et al. 2002). Only 44 per cent reported attending a follow-up clinic, while only 15 per cent had received a written record of their diagnosis and treatment for future reference. The effectiveness of standard follow-up surveillance in meeting some of the informational objectives of individual survivors is uncertain. Evidence from a small-scale study of 50 survivors in the UK found that only 10 per cent could name their cancer, 66 per cent were unable to name any of the drugs they had been given and only half could recall any discussions about the reasons for follow-up, although 62 per cent reported that they would like more information (Blacklay et al. 1998).

More specifically, several questionnaire surveys have indicated that survivors of childhood cancer experience worries about their reproductive capacity (Gray et al. 1992; Langeveld et al. 2004; Weigers et al. 1998). In one study around 60 per cent of the adult survivors of childhood cancer reported being unsure about whether their treatment for cancer had affected their fertility, and only half could recall ever having a discussion with a parent or health professional about the possible effects of treatment on their fertility status (Zebrack et al. 2004). Several women in Zebrack's study had experienced unplanned pregnancies because they had been informed that they were unlikely to be fertile and so had not used contraception. Conversely, some survivors were unnecessarily concerned about issues that were unlikely to present a threat to health, for example, several were concerned that they might pass on genetic problems to their future children, when there is little or no evidence that this is a significant risk.

Preparatory informational interventions and children's well-being

A rather different focus of the literature on communication comes from a body of research on the potential value of informational interventions to prepare children for specific medical procedures. In an early meta-analysis of studies of informational interventions to prepare acute and chronically ill children for a range of medical procedures, Saile et al. (1988) found evidence to suggest that informational interventions, including opportunities for verbal communication, play materials and videos, may be particularly helpful for children with chronic illnesses. There was also evidence to suggest that interventions prompting the active involvement of a child were more effective than those where the child remained mostly passive. However, only five of the 75 studies included in the review involved children with chronic illness who were being prepared for diagnostic and therapeutic procedures.

The difficulties of conducting syntheses of the evidence in this area are further illustrated by a recent Cochrane systematic review (Scott et al. 2001) which focused on informational interventions for children and adolescents with cancer. Of the 49 studies identified as potentially relevant, only six were judged eligible for inclusion in the review. The remaining studies were excluded because they did not meet the quality criteria for a Cochrane review, or employed designs other than randomized controlled trials (RCT). Clearly, there are a number of issues in assessing informational interventions that might limit the usefulness of evidence derived only from RCTs. In particular, the highly complex and sensitive nature of communicating with children with cancer makes it likely that a 'one size fits all' approach will rarely be appropriate and that interventions will almost certainly have to be tailored to children's needs, and adjusted to the different settings in which they are delivered. Moreover the focus on quantifiable outcomes such as knowledge and anxiety neglects the processes of meaning that are likely to be important in offering insights into children's experiences of information interventions. In the event, the review found modest evidence that interventions such as computer-assisted learning and school and social reintegration programmes could lead to improvements in children's knowledge and understanding of their condition, and to improved psychological, social and behavioural outcomes.

Problems with the 'information-giving' approach

While there are several important reasons for looking at what information children are given, this approach has a number of limitations. First, it tends to characterize children as the passive recipients of information, wholly dependent on parents to transmit information, as a sort of objective entity, to them. However, more sophisticated work has found that children with cancer are active in giving meaning to their illness and are able to work out many issues by gleaning information from the environment, but the sense that information is being concealed from them functions to create specific forms of restrictive social conditions. For example, terminally ill children were found to sense the gravity of their illness from the tone of overheard conversations, the emotional cues of those around them or from accidental disclosures, but were left unable to voice their concerns because of the 'mutual pretence' of that protectiveness that surrounded their illness (Bluebond-Langner 1974; Spinetta 1974). Second, the evidence on the links between information-giving practices and outcomes such as anxiety is weak and difficult to interpret. For example, demonstrating associations between parental reports of information-giving and specific outcomes is highly problematic.

Third, the literature on information-giving does not, as a rule, differentiate between different preferences for type and amount of information between children or between children's preferences at different stages of the illness, even though the adult literature has demonstrated not only that people do vary in what they want to know about cancer, but also that people's preferences vary along the trajectory of their illness and are not consistent over time (Leydon et al. 2000). Our qualitative work on communicating with children with cancer attests to the importance of discussions about procedures they were likely to face (Young et al. 2003). Almost all the children we interviewed reported finding information about the procedures they were to undergo to be extremely helpful and several spoke of the comfort that this information brought them, or of the worry and concern they felt they would experience if they knew little about what to expect. However, there were some limits to the depth or details that children wanted: almost all accounts contained references to the possibility that 'too much' information might be counterproductive and unnecessarily distressing. For example, a small number of children felt that information about certain aspects of treatment, particularly information about the amount of pain associated with certain procedures or other adverse outcomes of treatment, might exacerbate their anxiety and heighten their reluctance to undergo some procedures.

Most studies in the 'information-giving' approach have focused on the provision of information about diagnosis and prognosis, but it is clear that children's needs for information are more temporally variable and negotiated than this would imply. Beyond the crisis of the diagnosis, communication is likely to have important implications for the successful management of children's symptoms and the side effects of treatment (McGrath and Pitcher 2002). Woodgate et al. (2003) found that children viewed a worsening of symptoms as an indication that their illness was becoming more serious, and pointed to the importance of providing information about side-effects to prevent the unnecessary alarm that unexpected symptoms may generate. Children were also found to be less likely to report symptoms that were troubling, but which they considered to be a 'normal part of beating cancer'. Similarly, adolescents with a range of other chronic conditions rated information about day-to-day impact of the illness on their lives as being of equal importance to knowing about the condition and its management (Beresford and Sloper 2003).

In a small scale survey of information preferences of children with cancer aged 8–17 years, Ellis and Leventhal (1993) found that all children wanted to be told about their illness when it was diagnosed, and 62 per cent wanted to be told their diagnosis. Last and van Veldhuizen (1996) found that two-thirds of children wanted as much information as possible about their illness, the remaining one-third wanted minimal information, or expressed ambivalence about receiving detailed information. Blacklay et al. (1998) reported that a third of survivors expressed ambivalence or resistance to further information, and it is likely that a proportion of survivors may prefer to put the illness behind them and minimize their exposure to related issues. Similar feelings of ambivalence towards information have been reported in a study of chronically ill adolescents' experiences of communication (Beresford and Sloper 2003). These findings suggest there are likely to be important individual differences among children in their preferences and priorities for information. Indicating that the timing of information giving is another important consideration, Levenson et al. (1982) found that new patients and those in relapse were less likely to view additional information as helpful, suggesting that there may be times when patients may feel overwhelmed and prefer to avoid additional information. Taken together, this work appears to suggest that approaches that strongly advocate a policy of full and frank open communication are not necessarily in line with (all) children's preferences.

A further, and related, issue in the information-giving approach is the tendency to assume that information giving should take the same form, and that what works in one context will work in another. Children in our study (Young et al. 2003) talked in some detail about what they considered to be the most appropriate ways of supporting young patients to facilitate their communication and their assimilation of information. Most commented on the value of presenting information visually, and the usefulness of various props such as diagrams and models in helping them to understand health professionals' explanations. However, views were mixed about the common practice of using so-called child-friendly games and dolls to prepare children for procedures such as the insertion of Hickman lines. Though most children found these props helpful or did not comment in detail, a few were strongly critical of their use.

> *Interviewer*: I mean how was the Hickman line explained to you?

> *Child*: Not very, well they use like, they have a doll and that's quite babyish but that's how it was explained and they just kind of take out the blood from a doll and then they squeeze it back in. That's all, basically all they did. I wasn't really told that much about it ... it's for the younger children so they can explain it to them but it's not really good for me.
> (Female patient, aged 15, quoted in Young et al. 2003, unpublished)

> Yeah they explained to you, showed me the doll, but the doll's not very good because boys don't like dolls.
> (Male patient, aged 11, quoted in Young et al. 2003, unpublished)

Clearly, a few children considered these props to be unsuited to the level of explanation they required, or inappropriate to their gender, and encounters involving their use were experienced as humiliating and alienating. Such feelings could have major implications for the adequate management of children's care, for example, the 11-year-old boy quoted above went on to describe how the use of a doll in his preparation had 'put him off' having a Hickman line inserted, again demonstrating the inadequacy of 'one-size-fits-all' approaches to communication.

A final problem with the information-giving approach is its over-whelming tendency to assume that information should come from parents – most studies have focused on parents' reports of information giving, for example. In so doing, they fail adequately to problematize issues about *who* should communicate information to children with cancer and key issues about how the process should be managed, or to theorize why children *qua* patients should depend on their parents for information rather than doctors, or to acknowledge the complexity of parents' roles in the process.

The role of parents in communication

It is evident that there are a number of complex issues concerning parents as information-bearers. Our interviews with both children and parents suggest that most parents played an executive role in communication, actively managing what and how children are told about their illness, particularly at the time of diagnosis (Young et al. 2003). In this, parents' views and children's views on what children should be told may diverge. Ellis and Leventhal (1993), for example, found high levels of agreement between parents and children about the sharing of diagnostic information, but less agreement about sharing prognostic information. Only 30 per cent of parents listed prognostic information as one of the most important things their children should be told, compared with 62 per cent of children. There was also a marked divergence between children and parents about detailed discussion of side effects: while 77 per cent of children wanted to be told about all possible side effects, only 49 per cent of parents wanted their children to hear such information. Our study (Young et al. 2003) similarly found that some children wanted much more information than their parents seemed prepared to share with them. One way of explaining this phenomenon might be to argue, in line with the new social studies of childhood, that parents' communication behaviour rests on illegitimate assumptions about children's vulnerability and protection, and an oppressive social construction of children as incompetent in dealing with information about their own bodies. The empirical evidence, however, suggests that the explanations are rather more complex than this.

Our work (Young et al. 2003) suggests that the role parents adopt in communication is shaped by the emotional distress they experience in acute phases of the illness and by their concerns to manage their identity as strong and optimistic parents, a strategy they see as necessary to protect their child's well-being. This requirement is probably at its strongest around the time of the diagnosis and during subsequent illness or treatment crises, though it is also likely to become prominent in deliberations about disclosing the prognosis to children. Outside of situations that concern sensitive information or 'bad news', our work suggests that some parents may be willing to rescind a little on their executive role, and shift their alignment towards a partnership model, with child and parent roles becoming more equal and communication becoming more open. Evidence suggests that in making decisions about how to communicate with their children, parents are influenced by developmental considerations, and that these inform their ideas about what information it is appropriate to convey and about what emotions to display to children (Claflin and Barbarin 1991; Young et al. 2002; Young et al. 2003). That is not to say parents' approaches to communication are directly related to their child's age; indeed, though developmental considerations were prominent in the accounts of the parents in our studies, these were often differentially interpreted and utilized.

There is also evidence that parents use their own knowledge, and experience of their child, to determine what is appropriate. In our study (Young et al. 2003), some parents avoided discussion of sensitive topics with young children because they felt they lacked sufficient awareness to comprehend the information; other parents avoided the use of terms such as 'cancer' with children because they felt their child could understand the full significance of the term and would, therefore, become distressed. Parents' accounts are also influenced by their constructions of their children's unique character, including their emotional resilience or vulnerability. These expressions of uniqueness are a good deal more prominent in parents' accounts than they are in the literature. In addition, parents describe in some detail how their approach to communication is shaped by an overwhelming concern with ensuring that their child cooperates with treatment. Each of these considerations can either facilitate or constrain 'open' communication.

> As he said to be told, 'Oh you're going to be so ill and you're going to feel that' – I think that perhaps puts – would have put added pressure on him. Knowing those things were going to happen before they started. At least if you go in – a little bit in ignorance, then – you get through things maybe better – I – I don't know.
> (Parent of male patient, aged 15, quoted in Young et al. 2003 unpublished)

> And I think they did ask us, I don't remember that clearly, but I think someone did ask us, you know, how much do you want us to sort of say to [him], and you know we basically said we want to tell him, you know, everything really, and we want him, you know, if it hurts I think he needs to know. You can't sort of fob him off with anything.
> (Parent of male patient, aged 8, quoted in Young et al. unpublished)

It is also important to note that some parents may feel unable to handle discussing the illness with their child in the days and weeks after the diagnosis. Work by Eden et al. (1994) points to the difficulties that parents themselves experience in absorbing information in the early phases of the illness and how it can take some time before they feel emotionally ready to comprehend the news of their child's diagnosis. Talking about their experiences in trying to tell their child about the illness, the accounts of mothers in our studies underscore this finding (Young et al. 2002).

> We were too upset to be able to say it properly, I mean even trying to tell her that [she had poorly blood], we were in tears. So she obviously knew there was more than what we were telling her, because we were so upset. We weren't strong enough at that time to be able to tell her.
> (Mother of daughter, aged 10, quoted in Young et al. 2003).

Until parents feel ready, it may be unrealistic or counterproductive to expect them to handle full and frank discussions with their child, and we know little about the consequences for children of witnessing first hand their parents' sense of devastation as they try to talk about the illness with their children. It is also important for professionals to remain alert to the match between a child's information needs and preferences and their parents' approaches to information giving. A pronounced mismatch between these is likely to present difficulty for both children and parents and may have adverse consequences for the emotional well-being of the family more generally.

A further important, but neglected, influence on parents' ability to communicate with their children is, of course, their own experiences of information.

Parents' experiences of information

While most parents report being largely satisfied with information in the aftermath of their child's diagnosis (Sloper et al. 1996) several studies suggest that, if anything, too much information is provided for parents to absorb (Clarke and Fletcher 2003). After this initial period some feel that their questions remain unanswered and that opportunities to communicate with health professionals begin to diminish. This is a common theme in the literature on the parenting of children with chronic illnesses (Atkin and Ahmad 2000; Kvist et al. 1991; Young et al. 2002). For example, mothers in our study spoke about treatments being administered or changed without their knowledge, an issue that generated considerable distress for mothers and left them feeling undermined. Parents in Clarke and Fletcher's (2003) study identified problems with conflicting advice from health professionals, incorrect information, or information given in a confusing way.

The reasons for these difficulties are likely to be complex but evidence indicates that while parents find information about their child's condition to be a great help in caring for them, professionals seriously underestimate parents' desire for information (James et al. 2002; Perrin et al. 2000). Parents may sometimes be reluctant to voice their questions even though they would like further information because they are fearful of hearing 'bad news'. McGrath and Pitcher (2002) found that some parents were reluctant to raise their concerns about the behavioural side effects of some treatments because they feel it is their responsibility to deal with such matters themselves. They also worried that they might be creating a nuisance by asking 'too many questions', or that they might be placing unreasonable burdens on staff who were perceived to be 'very busy'. These feeling may intensify later in the illness with parents' increased sense of responsibility for monitoring their children's health and securing the well-being of their children.

> I mean we were given quite a lot of information right at the beginning when [my son] was first diagnosed ... and then I feel it kind of tapered off ... I mean you ask questions and people are happy to answer those questions but ... it's not always a good time in clinic or when [my son] is having treatment to ask questions, obviously people are busy ... And once or twice [my son] has had a kind of reaction to something ... and nobody had sort of said, 'Oh this might happen.' And when I got him over [to the hospital] it was very calmly explained to me that this is something that happens quite a lot. And I thought okay that's fine, that's stopped me from worrying but I'd just driven sort of 40 minutes from [home] with a very sick little boy ... If that had been explained to me I could have dealt with that here.
>
> (Mother of male patient, aged 6, cited in Young et al. 2002: 1843)

Parents in some studies have also identified difficulties in their relationships with health professionals, particularly a lack of staff continuity during the course of their child's treatment, or insensitive communication (Clarke and Fletcher 2003; Kvist et al. 1991; Patterson et al. 2004). For families of children who experienced a protracted diagnosis, difficulties may continue into the treatment phase and beyond (Eiser et al. 1995; Swallow and Jacoby 2001).

The consultation

This work explains why it may be difficult for parents to perfectly align their information giving with children's preferences, but it does not explain why parents find themselves in the role of information bearers, rather than, for example, professionals. The answers to why parents come to assume this role are likely to be found in ethnographic work observing parent–child interactions in a range of settings, and in detailed similar work investigating consultations. However, with the exception of Bluebond-Langner's (1978) ethnographic participant observations of paediatric oncology wards, very little research appears to have directly examined child–parent–professional encounters in paediatric oncology settings. Therefore, we know little about how consultations involving children are conducted, and how meanings and roles are constructed and negotiated in these settings. Evidence from other healthcare contexts suggests that children frequently appear to be marginalized in consultations, and that this is particularly evident in the case of younger children.

Child, parent, professional communication outside childhood cancer

Some of the most important work in developing the sociology of patient–professional interaction (for example, Silverman 1987; Strong 1979) was based on observations of paediatric consultations. This work was hugely important in identifying the ways in which roles, identities and norms are negotiated in medical consultations, for example, through rules of etiquette and ceremonial forms, and we have already discussed many of these in relation to parents' attempts to obtain a diagnosis of childhood cancer in Chapter 2. Ironically, although both of these studies involved consultations about children, neither included a sustained specific focus on children's roles, though both showed the ways in which children appear to have a non-participant status in consultations. Strong, for example, identified that there was an unwillingness to admit children to any relationship of equality in the doctor–child–parent relationship, but our knowledge of how consultations have moved on since his study more than 25 years ago remains lamentably lacking (Gabe et al. 2004).

Evidence thus far does suggest that children continue to be heard, or speak, little in medical consultations. In a study of hospital-based outpatient consultations for children with a variety of conditions, van Dulman (1998) found that paediatricians directed a quarter of their medical questions at children, but only one tenth of the medical information they provided was directed at children. Children's contributions to the consultation accounted for only 4 per cent of utterances, compared with 37 per cent and 59 per cent for parents and paediatricians respectively. Parents frequently answered questions that were directed at children, and children's participation was limited largely to social talk and laughter, and to providing of some information on the experience of symptoms. More recent research by van Dulman (2004) suggests that paediatricians still tend to exclude child patients and to experience difficulties in conducting 'true multi-party talk' with parents and children.

Developing some of the themes from van Dulman's (2004) study, Tates and Meeuwesen's (2000) work on turn taking in general practice encounters found that children's involvement in communication was limited by adult turn-taking behaviour. Parents appeared to exclude children by speaking in response to more than half of the turns that GPs explicitly directed to children. Age was a strong predictor of children's involvement in communication; older children were more likely to speak up in response to GP utterances that had been directed at parents, and GPs were also more likely to address older children directly and to allocate fewer turns to parents. By contrast, parents' turn taking did not seem to vary according to child age.

Tates et al. (2002) explain the patterns of communication observed in interactions with child patients in terms of the roles and identities that participants bring to the interaction, and how participants work collaboratively to 'co-construct' or negotiate the course of the consultation. They suggest that parents take responsibility for speaking for their child as matters of child health and well-being are a fundamental part of the parenting role and identity, and note that patterns of communication early in the consultation seem to structure what happens subsequently. Even where a GP initially invites a child to participate in formulating the reason for the consultation, in most cases it is the doctor and parent who exclusively accomplish the information exchanges around diagnosis and treatment, while the child occupies the role of a 'withdrawn bystander' in her own consultation. According to Tates et al. (2002), the family doctors in their study appeared to accept their roles, and as the consultation progressed they focused their alignment increasingly with the parents. Children very rarely challenge these alignments, and while GPs have scope to refocus the course of the consultation by inviting children's comments, they very rarely make use of this option. Tates et al. (2002) suggest that the low degree of child participation in child–parent–doctor encounters should not be viewed as a sign of children's incompetence, but rather as a feature of children's and adults' roles and linguistic practices, and how these operate to limit children's active participation in communication.

Silverman et al.'s (1998) analysis of turn-taking in hospital clinics for adolescents finds that young people rarely speak, but shows that they often do not speak even when the turn taking specifically invites them to do so, particularly in situations where advice is being given. Silverman et al. draw the interesting conclusion that it is possible to consider the non-responses of young people as accomplishments in their own right, concluding that 'By no means is the silent child not a competent child' (p. 239). This insight lends a rather different perspective to the rather stark findings from other studies of apparent non-participation by children, by showing that children may in fact use their silence strategically. Our own work (Young et al. 2003), though not based on direct observations of consultations, also suggests that children can be strategic in their behaviour in the consultation and outside it, use parents and others as resources, a point we develop below.

Children's views and experiences of the consultation in the context of childhood cancer

In addition to this work on turn taking, it is also important to understand the perspectives of the various parties within these encounters. A survey of people aged 11–20 by Levenson et al. (1982) suggests that consultations with health professionals are highly important to children. While very few young people indicated a preference for written or audiovisual materials as their main source of information, close to 70 per cent preferred their information needs to be met through discussions with health professionals, though many also wanted their parents to be included in these discussions. However, there is some evidence that children with cancer have unsatisfactory interactions with health professionals. In a small qualitative study of 10 children and their families Inman (1991) characterized consultant interactions with children in paediatric oncology clinics as short, fragmented, absent-minded and frequently interrupted by adults, or by the requirement to perform examinations of children.

The accounts of some young people in our study of experiences of communication about childhood cancer (Young et al. 2003) suggest that children feel some of their priorities are of little interest to professionals, and that they therefore suppress them.

> *Young person*: I probably wouldn't ask what something meant . . . just 'cos I might look stupid . . . [I] don't really mind that much about all the facts, I don't want to know that much about all that. I just want to know all the silly things, like.
>
> *Interviewer*: Silly things?
>
> *Young person*: Well, not like important things, like your hair and school and things like that.
>
> *Interviewer*: And you don't think they're important or . . .?
>
> *Young person*: Well I do but they probably don't because it's not like medical stuff.
>
> (Female patient, aged 15, quoted in Young et al. 2003: 307).

There is also some evidence that children may have difficulties in articulating or verbalizing what they want to say. For example, a possible barrier to communication for the younger children in Woodgate and Degner's study (2003) was their tendency to experience symptoms as overall feelings states, for example, 'feeling yucky'. Some children had difficulty or were uninterested in discussing symptoms when these were disaggregated as discrete side effects or singular states, suggesting that appropriate conceptual frames are needed to help children to discuss their symptoms.

Children have, of course, to negotiate their parents' presence in the consultation as well as their relationship with professionals. Some work has found that children find some elements of their parents' role help to facilitate communication with health professionals, for example, by giving children the confidence to ask questions (Beresford and Sloper 2003). Children in our study (Young et al. 2003) generally welcomed their parents' involvement, but expressed unease with some aspects of their parents' role, which was sometimes seen as an unwelcome constraint on access to information about their illness. Some children expressed disquiet at the perceived disparities between how much information they themselves were given and how much their parents had been given. This finding resonates with the work of other researchers which indicated that while three-quarters of parents wanted the option to discuss issues that they did not want their child to know about, less than 20 per cent of children agreed such discussions should occur (Ellis and Leventhal 1993).

Our work indicates that the presence of parents in the consultation can leave children feeling feel marginalized and lead to difficulties for children in understanding what health professionals were saying.

> I think sometimes they talk to both of us, but sometimes they – I find they do just talk to mum and I, just, 'Hello? I'm sitting here' ... especially with the consultants, it's just talking to mum. You know, um, 'Hello?'
> (Male patient, aged 15, quoted in Young et al. 2003: 307)

> Well, for starters, like when they were talking about what was happening and that, they used to like talk to my mum and dad, they didn't like exactly talk to me. So I didn't exactly know what was going on 'cos they were just like talking to my mum, even though I was still in the same room. It was difficult 'cos they weren't exactly talking to me about what was happening.
> (Female patient, aged 10, quoted in Young et al. 2003 unpublished)

While parents' roles in communication could sometimes cause difficulties, this does not mean that children would have preferred their parents to adopt an arm's-length role in communication. Above all, young people's preferences for their parents' involvement were fluid and context dependent. Reflecting work with adult patients on awareness contexts (Timmermans 1994), almost all the young people in our study at times embraced or even actively cultivated their parents' role as "buffers" to limit their exposure to information.

> But I felt that what [the doctor] was going to speak to my mum and dad about, I didn't really need to know about it that much. Just something for mum and dad to be concerned about, I didn't really need to know about it so – I thought that was the best thing.
> (Male patient, aged 15, quoted in Young et al. 2003: 307)

This strategic use of parents extended to four distinct roles that children and young people see for their parents in communication:

- *facilitators of communication between health professionals and them-selves*: for example, parents' presence in consultations sometimes gave children the confidence to ask questions;
- *envoys*: for example, when the young people briefed their parents to seek information on their behalf;
- *communication buffers*: for example, when the young people used their parents to shield them from the burden of answering questions
- *human databases*: when parents acted as cataloguers and repositories of information about the illness;
- *communication brokers*: when parents customized, clarified, or re-iterated information so that the children could better assimilate what health professionals had said.

The child–professional relationship

Attention to roles and relationships in communication reminds us that communication serves functions that go far beyond the content of the information exchanged in particular encounters and that attention needs to be given to the processes of meaning construction. Like adults, children need to be able to trust their health professionals and develop a relationship with them, yet virtually no research on communication in childhood cancer has explored the child–professional relationship and particularly how these relationships vary with different professionals.

A prominent theme in accounts of the children in our interviews was the importance of 'getting to know' or developing a familiarity with the different professionals involved in their care (Young et al. 2003). Familiarity helped children to access information. For example, it helped children select professionals whom they felt were best placed to answer questions on particular issues and lent them confidence in voicing those questions. More importantly, however, 'getting to know' was regarded as critical for children in being able to 'trust' health professionals and develop a relationship with them.

> Because you need – you need the reassurance of the people that are going to be – with you throughout it. You need to know who these people are.
> (Male patient, aged 15, quoted from Young et al. 2003, unpublished)

> Because if they don't get to know their doctor, then they might suffer a bit, from – um – what they think might happen. And if they don't

get to know their doctor then they might actually start to get a bit worried about what's going to happen to them.
(Male patient, aged 8, quoted from Young et al. 2003 unpublished)

Communication creates a space through which children can begin to establish a relationship with, and through which they can begin to trust, health professionals. However, we have seen how communication is managed or conducted, and the role that parents and professionals adopt can leave children feeling marginalized and act a barrier to establishing such a relationship. Another possible barrier is children's awareness of their status and the relative powerlessness of this position. Beresford and Sloper (2003) found that perceptions of high doctor status could be powerful inhibitors of communication, particularly for younger adolescents and those who lacked confidence. These status differences are undoubtedly a further obstacle to children's sense that they can directly call on their health professionals as a source of support, and not simply access them vicariously through their parents.

Conclusions

Much research on communication in childhood cancer has tended to focus on quantifying or cataloguing the openness of communication, and attempting to examine the implications of particular approaches or strategies on children's well-being. Attempts to quantify and categorize the information given to children suggest an overall trend to more detailed information-giving in recent years. These studies also suggest that younger children are given less information than older children. While these issues are of considerable importance, rather less attention has been given to communication as a social and emotional process, and the complexities of managing the three-way relationship between children, parents and professionals. We have seen that the way in which communication is managed, and role that parents adopt in the consultation, can leave children marginalized and isolated, but also that children may choose strategically to use their parents as communication resources and that there is a need to see communication processes as fluid and continually negotiated.

We wish to be clear that we are not making an argument for or against open communication; only that such arguments be based on sound evidence. Issues of development and concerns about children's competence have tended to dominate the research agenda and one consequence appears to be that little research has investigated children's preferences and priorities. Little work has also investigated the match between the preferences of children and those of their parents, or indeed what happens in situations where these are mismatched. Paradoxically, and perhaps reflecting the dichotomized thinking of the 'telling versus not telling' debates, there is a strong push in some work on communication to strongly advocate for a policy of open communication with children. Such approaches need to take account of the role of the parents, and if adopted rigidly or too literally, may conflict with the priorities and preferences of children and families. Clearly too, the ways that parents experience communication require specific attention; as we have made clear in earlier chapters, parents are participants in their child's experience of cancer, and have to assume multiple demanding roles and undertake many different types of labour in the fulfilment of these.

7 Shared decision making in childhood cancer

Children with cancer and their families are confronted with numerous decisions during the course of their treatment and subsequently. The nature and significance of decisions vary along the course of the treatment, and raise different types of issues. Some decisions may need to be taken before treatment commences, including whether to participate in a trial or other research, whether to store sperm or eggs, or whether to undertake surgery. Particularly difficult issues may arise in cases of relapsed or refractory disease, where decisions need to be made about bone-marrow transplants, palliative chemotherapy, and further treatment. Every day, more minor decisions will need to be made: who is to be present during lumbar punctures, whether to use sedation during some procedures, whether to agree to be examined, when to return to school and social activities, whether to go swimming. We have tried to illustrate the range of types of decision in a series of case studies (1–6) in this chapter.

Box 7.1 Case studies

Case study 1
Tariq is 7 years old and hates lumbar punctures. He wants to refuse to have one although doctors have explained to him that a lumbar puncture is vital to determine the stage of his disease and what his next treatment should comprise. His doctors and parents agree that the lumbar puncture must go ahead.

Case study 2
Chloe is 8 years old and about to undergo treatment which is likely to destroy her ova. Her doctors have discussed with her parents and herself the possibility of a procedure to remove and store some eggs using freezing techniques. It is uncertain whether this procedure would restore her fertility later in life and doctors have stressed that it is still experimental. Her mother is keen to go ahead with the operation to remove the eggs, but her father disagrees, saying that Chloe has put up with enough and should not be put through another procedure under general anaesthetic, which she hates, if it is not necessary to save her life. Chloe herself says she is fed up of hospitals and does not want to discuss the matter.

Case study 3

Mark is a 10-year-old routinely described as exceptionally mature and intelligent. Chemotherapy for his ALL failed and he had a bone marrow transplant from his only sibling (a sister aged 4) which he found very traumatic. This also failed and the option of a second bone marrow transplant has been offered, but he is aware that the chances of success are very slim. He does not want to put himself or his sister through the procedure and has asked to have palliative chemotherapy aimed at improving his quality of life before he dies. His father, who is divorced from the mother but has parental responsibility, is distraught and insisting the second bone marrow transplant goes ahead. His mother says the decision is Mark's to make. Doctors say the decision must be made by the family, though they warn that this procedure is rarely successful.

Case study 4

Marco, a 15-year-old male, was a keen footballer until diagnosed with osteosarcoma (originating in his right ankle) two months ago. All of his friends are footballers and Marco had dreamt of playing professionally. The doctors have explained that Marco's only chance of survival is amputation of his right leg below the knee, because the cancer is highly aggressive and is likely to spread. Marco refuses, saying that he would rather die than have his leg cut off.

Case study 5

A 12-year-old, Elaine, had some difficulties in settling into secondary school. She then became 'best' friends with Amirta and the two were inseparable until Elaine was diagnosed with ALL and admitted to hospital for lengthy blocks of treatment. Amirta has been to visit Elaine in hospital but Elaine has been agonized that Amirta will become fed up, forget about her, and make other friends. Amirta is having a big party for her 13th birthday in a local leisure centre. There will be 200 people there. Although Elaine is now at home following a block of treatment, her doctors have advised her not to attend as she is currently neutropenic (low in cells that fight bacterial infection) and vulnerable to infection. Elaine is determined not to miss the party.

Case study 6

Paul, aged 17, completed treatment for cancer last year and is scheduled for review follow-up visits to the clinic every three months. He refuses to attend. He says he wants to forget he ever had cancer, and that if his employers find out he is under medical care he will be fired as he claimed in his job application to be in good health. He also has not told his partner, who is pregnant, that he once had cancer.

An important context for our discussion of decision making is that, as we have described earlier in this book, successful treatment of childhood cancer (where success is defined in terms of survival) depends crucially on rigid adherence to standardized protocols. When an attempt is made to depart from these, very serious disagreements can arise. Sometimes children wish to make choices that adults contest. The most frequent (probably daily) scenario concerns children wishing to refuse treatment (Stokes and Drake-Lee 1998; Tomlinson 2004) though the refusals are at different levels, from the younger child wishing to refuse a procedure (case study 1) to the young person wishing to reject treatment altogether (case studies 3, 4 and 6). Other situations involve children and young people not wishing to comply with medical advice (case study 5).

The literature on children's involvement in decision making has indeed been almost entirely preoccupied with debates on children's *rights* to consent, and to a lesser extent on their *right* to participate in decisions. This contrasts with the large adult literature on 'patient partnership' (Charles et al. 1999b) which has focused on sharing of information and decision making, as well as the issues of *quality* of consent (though there is also a literature on adult rights, for example in relation to capacity). As we shall argue, this focus on children's rights – a normative question – has led to a neglect of empirical and theoretical questions about how children with cancer and their families are involved in decision making, how to explain current practices and, crucially, preferences in relation to decision making. We will discuss the limited evidence on shared decision making in relation to childhood cancer, but will foreground this with a discussion of the debates about rights. These complex and wide-ranging debates about decision making occur across the boundaries of law, ethics, social science and philosophy, concern issues of the moral and political status of children, and rest crucially on notions of ideology, social construction, rights, duties and competence as well as ethical principles. The issues are different depending on the age of the child – as Brazier (2003) notes, there are differences between situations where everyone agrees that a child is too young to make decisions for him- or herself, and the vexed issues surrounding young people.

Law on consent

Children's rights to participation in decision making and authority over consent are covered by a complex combination of statute and case law. We have space here to offer only a brief overview of the area, and it is beyond the scope of this chapter to address complex legal issues such as those raised by case study 2 (Chloe) in relation to the Human Fertilisation and Embryology Act (1990).

The ethical principle that individuals have a right to self-determination and are entitled to have their autonomy respected finds its expression in law through the notion of consent (Kennedy and Grubb 2000). A doctor is not entitled to treat a patient without the consent of someone authorized to give it. However, for those aged under 18 years, the right to give or withhold consent is more limited. In law, a person who has not yet attained the age of 18 years is deemed 'a minor', and the role of those with 'parental responsibility' becomes important. A person with parental responsibility may be the child's mother, married father, or – under the Children Act (1989) – unmarried father (with agreement with the mother or where a court order has been made giving him that power), a person holding a residence order or a local authority (McHale and Tingle 2001). For simplicity, we will refer to people with parental responsibility as 'parents'.

The principle that children should be consulted, informed and involved in decisions affecting them, but lack the final authority over decisions, is enshrined in the UN Convention of the Rights of the Child (UNCRC). Ratified by the UK (in 1991) and most other countries worldwide, this instrument incorporates the full range of human rights – civil, political, economic, social and cultural. The UNCRC includes a number of provisions aimed at securing children's welfare and protection rights, but several provisions reflect children's rights to participation, including, in particular, Article 12. This states that children have the right to participate in decision-making processes that may be relevant in their lives, and to influence decisions taken in their regard. While the Convention confirms that children have the right to express their views and have their views taken seriously, it does not state that children's views are the only ones to be considered. The guiding principle of the UNCRC is that the 'best interests' of the child must be promoted, but it is clear that differences of opinion between parents, children and professionals about the 'best interests' of the child will sometimes need to be resolved. The UNCRC explicitly states that children have a responsibility to respect the rights of others, including and especially those of their parents, and emphasizes the need to recognize children's 'evolving capacities':

> Respecting children's views means that such views should not be ignored; it does not mean that children's opinions should be automatically endorsed. Expressing an opinion is not the same as taking a decision, but it implies the ability to influence decisions.
>
> (http://www.unicef.org/crc/crc.htm)

What reaches courts, of course, are disputes. Disputes can arise in various ways: when a person under 18 refuses to consent to a treatment that parents and medical staff consider to be in his or her best interests; when parents refuse to consent; or when both child and parent refuse to consent.

Under current English law, under Section 8 of the Family Law Reform Act (1969), people aged 16 or 17 are entitled to give consent to surgical, medical and dental treatment. Famously, the Gillick case (*Gillick v. West Norfolk and Wisbech Area Health Authority [1985] 3 ER 402*) allowed that children under the age of 16 may also have competence to consent to treatment if they have 'sufficient maturity' to do so. Whether a child is deemed to have this maturity is a decision-relative test (McHale and Gallagher 2003), and, therefore, varies from situation to situation – a child may be deemed competent to give consent to some procedures (such as the insertion of a Hickman line) but not to others (for example, an amputation).

Although 'competent' young people – whether under or over 16 years – may consent to treatment, their ability to refuse treatment is more restricted (Brazier 2003; Kennedy and Grubb 2000). The Court of Appeal has established that in a situation in which a competent adolescent refuses treatment, consent may be given either by a person with parental responsibility or by the court (McHale and Gallagher 2003). Unlike adults, therefore, the refusal of a competent person under 18 may be overruled, though the courts have indicated that the child's views are an important consideration and that this importance increases with the age and maturity of the child (for example, *Re W (A Minor) (Medical Treatment) [1992] 4 All ER 627*) Indeed, the Children's Act (1989) and accompanying guidance and regulations place considerable emphasis on taking account of the child's views, although, as McHale et al. (1997) comment, it contains very little about the rights of minors to make independent decisions about medical treatment.

McHale and Gallagher (2003) have considered whether the Human Rights Act (1998) would make a difference to cases where young people refuse to consent. They point out that a number of European Convention on Human Rights Convention rights are potentially applicable, but conclude that how the courts will proceed is uncertain. They suggest that it is likely that judicial approaches will be cautious and favour adherence with medical advice in the case of very young children, but the application to older children is more questionable. Parents as well as children may disagree with medical advice. In the past, parental objections to clinical procedures have generally been overridden by the courts (McHale and Gallagher 2003). For example, when the parents' refusal to consent to blood transfusion is deemed to endanger the child's life, the courts have invariably given leave for it to be administered (Downie 1999). Many of these cases have involved objections on religious grounds. Although courts may overrule parents who do not agree with what medical opinion deems to be in the best interests of the child, Strasbourg case law now provides a stronger means for parents to challenge any perceived lack of involvement in the decision-making process (Hagger 2004). Again, there is a possibility of litigation regarding the application of Article 8 of the Human Rights Act (1998), concerning the right to privacy of home and family life, in cases where courts seek to overrule parents' decisions regarding the treatment of their child. McHale and Tingle (2001) suggest that consideration of the child's welfare is likely to remain paramount, and the successful use of Article 8 is somewhat unlikely.

It is clear that, although increasingly concerned to take children's wishes and preferences into account whenever possible (Roche 1996), the law continues, nonetheless, to limit their rights to complete autonomy, and, at least for the present, provides recourse for those who believe they are acting in a child's best interests in making decisions about serious matters. The recognition of agency implied by the UN Convention and in the Children Act is, therefore, argued by some working within the 'new' social studies of childhood to be little more than rhetoric (James and James 2001b).

Children's rights to participation

As Gabe et al. (2004) and Dingwall (1994) note, the formal legal environment acts as a powerful constraint on the possibilities of interactions between health professionals and patients. James and James (2004) argue that the law is also important because of the ways in which it contributes to the production, regulation and reproduction of childhood over time: it represents a highly specialized system of thinking about social realities and their regulation, and powerfully embodies discourses about childhood. Legal codes, James and James (2004) propose, work to institutionalize childhood by defining key aspects of the relationship between adults and children. While we agree that the law certainly provides an important framework within which social actors function, we argue also that an examination of law on consent provides only a very limited understanding of how decision making in childhood cancer operates in practice, and that discussion of specific legal cases has skewed the debate in the direction of extreme and unusual cases at the expense of a more measured debate (and empirical investigation) about the routine and everyday management of decision making.

Though the law may act as an important constraint, most decisions in childhood cancer are made informally and are negotiated within particular forms of social relations. For example, no formal process of consent will be involved in the case of the girl who wants to go swimming at her friend's party (case study 5), and the 7-year-old who does not want a lumbar puncture (case study 1) is likely to be managed by explanation, soothing, comfort and reassurance rather than by a protracted negotiation about who has the final say. We suggest that much of the debate about children's rights to participation have focused on formal rights, at the expense of an empirical and theoretical exploration of how children's participation is managed informally and what the consequences of different models of decision making might be.

Before we develop this argument, however, any discussion about decision making in childhood cancer must be located within wider debates about children's rights. Generally speaking, three different types of rights can be distinguished: first, 'welfare' or 'provision' rights, which offer children certain entitlements to education, food and shelter; second 'protection' rights, which entitle children to freedom from violence and cruelty, and third, rights of agency, which entitle children to participation. Lowden (2002) drawing on work by the UK National Children's Bureau, distinguishes three different approaches to children's rights to participation: protectionist, liberationist and pragmatist. The protectionist approach sees adults as guardians and defenders of children, and assumes that children should be protected from making decisions for their own good. The pragmatist approach attempts to achieve a balance between protectionism and liberationist ideas, and is explicit about the need both to value children's knowledge, insight and preferences, and also to protect children from making decisions that might have serious adverse consequences. The liberationist approach characterizes children as oppressed and prevented from achieving autonomy by unwarranted assumptions about their competence. Much of the debate arises because of the inherent potential for conflict between rights of protection and provision, and rights of participation.

The protectionist approach

The new social studies of childhood argues that childhood has been constructed as a 'protectionist experience' (Jenks 1996a), where rights to protection are assumed, but rights to autonomy and participation tend to be denied. Those working within a protectionist approach argue that children are inherently vulnerable, that their most prominent rights are to protection and provision, and that rights to participation should not be instituted without demonstration of the benefits for children. Brighouse (2002), for example, claims that granting children rights is not the appropriate means to protect their interests. He points out that the immediate agency interests of children differ greatly from those of adults (that is, their own future agency interests). He also points to children's lack of competence, arguing that children (particularly younger ones) lack key experiences and conceptions that are essential for an understanding of one's interests as an adult. Ben-porath (2003) makes a similar argument, seeking to protect children from the unwanted consequences of having to make decisions, and proposing that society should, therefore, prefer protective paternalism, and derive from this approach specific institutional obligations, including obligations on the part of the family, the welfare and medical institutions, and the education system. The protectionist approach might, therefore, be summarized as seeking to limit children's rights to participation in decision making, and to consent, in the interests of their welfare rights.

The pragmatist approach

Most attempts to apply principles of involvement in decision making by children in the area of healthcare have adopted a pragmatist approach, where children are explicitly encouraged to participate and *have a say*, but stop short of offering children final authority or granting children rights to full self-determination. This approach is evident in most professional statements on the involvement of children. The American Academy of Pediatrics (1995) proposes that parents and doctors should not exclude children and adolescents from decision making without persuasive reasons. The Royal College of Paediatrics and Child Health (2000) recommends that children should be addressed in their own right, and that competent children be given information relevant to their health, and be involved in making decisions. The British Medical Association (2001) similarly emphasizes the need to inform and involve children, and counsels that age is not the most important factor in whether children may make their own decisions. Within childhood cancer specifically, recent guidelines on informed consent urge doctors to share information with children and to facilitate the involvement of children in decision making (Spinetta et al. 2003), but again have not proposed to offer children rights to full self-determination.

The liberationist approach

The caution evident in the protectionist and pragmatist approaches, however, is challenged by those working at the liberationist end of the spectrum, driven by an attempt to recognize the rights of children and young people as autonomous moral agents who are capable of making competent and rational choices. The debate about children's rights to participation has been raging since the 1970s, which saw a number of manifestos proclaiming the need for children to be liberated. Archard (1993) summarizes the basic claims of the children's liberationists as follows: first, the modern separation of the child and adult worlds constitutes unwarranted and reinforced discrimination resting on a false ideology of 'childishness', and second, children are entitled to all the rights and privileges of adults. Founded on the idea that each person is an autonomous individual, the liberationist position argues that it is manifestly unfair to distribute rights on the basis of age.

Within the broad church of those working within a 'liberationist' paradigm of children's rights, a number of different positions can be discerned, from those in the 'youth rights' movement associated with the work of Holt (1975), who demand the right to total legal and financial rights for children, to those at the more pragmatist end of the spectrum. The liberationist approach is, of course, closely allied to the social constructionist approach to childhood, and some (for example, Freeman 1998) have explicitly sought to integrate their agendas further: it is clearly only a short step from the identification of children's *ontological* agency to the promotion of children's *moral* agency. As we explained in Chapter 1, the social constructionist approach challenges attempts to render features of childhood as 'natural' or 'inherent' to children, instead seeing attributes such as competence or capacity as socially constructed characteristics. Jenks (1996a) for example, argues that dominant psychological and paediatric theories of child development in westernized societies render childhood an essentially protectionist experience; children find their lives shaped by statutes that are founded on ideological discourses about childhood that see them as not fully rational, and as lacking in the insight and wisdom to know their own best interests.

The 'best interests' problem

A key issue in debates around the wisdom of involving children in decision making and their authority of consent has concerned the problem of 'best interests', which underlies the exercise of beneficence on behalf of others. Those working within the new social studies of childhood argue that the assumption that adults know best is founded on an illegitimate view of children as incompetent, irresponsible and lacking in capacity, pointing to evidence that the meanings given to children's 'best interests' are culturally specific (Solberg 1997). It is further noted that families may not necessarily serve the best interests of their children (Butler 1996), and as we noted earlier in this book, some research is beginning to emerge to suggest that the views of children, parents and physicians may not always converge. In some of the examples illustrated in our case studies at the start of this chapter, it is not at all clear how 'best interests' can be determined. Indeed, as Archard and Macleod (2002) point out, 'it no longer seems possible to posit a simple harmony between the interests of children and those charged with the responsibility of rearing them, such that the exercise of authority over children during their development of maturity can be viewed as a fairly straightforward matter'.

Those working within pragmatist and protectionist approaches propose that children need to be protected from having final authority over (at least some) decisions that might affect their welfare. Those working within the liberationist tradition contend that the welfare rights of children are invoked to serve as forms of control. A common tendency within the liberationist approach is to portray adults as a dominant and oppressive group who suppress (or even brutally repress) the legitimate claims of children to self-determination.

> Some adults argue that if you let children decide for themselves, they
> will refuse medical treatment, because they are too ignorant, foolish
> and inexperienced to know their own best interests. Yet the right to
> self-determination is the key to all rights. You can talk about re-
> sources, care and protection under the heading of children's welfare
> or interests, but do not need to use rights language to promote these
> benefits. The right to choose is a crucial part of being a right holder.
> Alice Miller, the Swiss psychoanalyst, has shown that centuries of
> harsh, even cruel, child-rearing illustrate differences between adults'
> ideas of 'care', 'protection', what is 'right for children', versus chil-
> dren's rights to choose how they would live.
>
> (Alderson 1993b: 13)

Within this perspective, children are denied participation rights because
of a reluctance to give them credit for being what Mayall (1994b: 8) describes
as 'moral interpreters of the worlds they engage with, capable of participating
in shared decisions on important topics'.

Alderson (1994) adopts the position that the failure to allow competent
children to make decisions amounts to discrimination against a minority
group by an oppressive adult majority, proposing (Alderson 2000) that the
dominance of professional and public beliefs about childhood by Piaget's
work and myths has convinced many adults that they must protect and
control children without needing to consult them. She argues that the most
powerful way to justify coercion '. . . is to deny that children can be competent, and to align adult reason with force; children's resistance is then seen as
mindless "self-destruction", to be overridden by rational adults' (Alderson
1994). James and James (2004) argue that if a child judged to be Gillick
competent can be overruled, then this involves a failure to respect the pro-
position that a competent child can take responsibility for herself, and a lack
of respect for a child's right to self-determination and bodily integrity.

Within this tradition, attempts to use children's welfare as a reason for
overruling them are seen simply as a convenient way to excuse the exercise of
power and to deny children rights (Lansdown 1994). Oakley (1994) similarly
suggests that the language of 'best interests' is a philosophy of exclusion and
control dressed up as protection, and dependent on the notion that those
who are protected must be so because they are deemed incapable of looking
after themselves. The construct of vulnerability that underlies many of the
protectionist policies towards children is argued to be flawed, and Roche
(1999) makes the case that many of the sociobiological assumptions concerning reasoning and moral capacity that once denied women agency now
prevail in relation to children:

> If older children are no longer to be distinguished from adults on the basis of a presumed intellectual and cognitive inferiority, on what basis can we routinely exclude children from full participation in the life of the community to which they belong? How can we justify practices, which presuppose the non-participation of children?
>
> (Roche 1999: 482)

In pointing to the ways in which the law, and social discourses more generally, tend to illegitimately disadvantage children, James and James (2004) argue that children are, in fact, required to demonstrate *greater* competence than adults in cases where they wish to exercise self-determination. They discuss in some detail the case of a 15-year-old Jehovah's Witness with leukaemia who was refusing blood transfusions and wished to be allowed to die (*Re E (a minor) (wardship: medical treatment) [1993] 1 FLR 386*). In this case the young person was overruled by the court on the grounds that he was not Gillick competent because did not have sufficient comprehension of the pain, suffering and fear that would be involved in his death and, therefore, did not have a full understanding within the meaning of Gillick. James and James (2004) argue that having insight into one's own death is an exceeding high standard of competence, and that the law of competence is being distorted to avoid the consequences of a child's decision. They point out that on achieving the age of 18 this young person exercised his right as an adult to refuse treatment and subsequently died, and emphasize the arbitrariness involved in preventing someone aged just under 18 years to make a decision while allowing someone just over this age to make one. In this way, they claim that the boundaries that separate adulthood and childhood are artificial and illegitimate.

Problems with the liberationist approach

The liberationist position argues that any competent child should be involved in decision making and have the right to consent to or refuse treatment, and locates the failure to award such rights in power relations between children and adults. There are, however, a number of problems in applying the liberationist position, its claims, and its aspirations to childhood cancer.

First, the argument that social constructions of children (especially very ill children) as vulnerable and having age-related competencies and capacities are founded on 'false' ideologies inspired by developmental psychology is difficult to sustain. The claim that Piagetian discourses have somehow pervaded everyday practices and professional and legal discourses cannot easily be substantiated, and it gives little credit to adults for their own agency in giving meaning to the experiences of children they interact with. It is entirely possible that assumptions about children are in fact based on observations of children in everyday life, recognitions that children of different ages do perceive and behave differently, and insights into the vulnerability of children in extremely difficult and demanding circumstances.

Perhaps the most important critique, because of its practical consequences, centres on the role given to competence in the liberationist position. Central to the liberationist approach is the argument that the decision of a competent person should be respected, as to do otherwise denies a moral right to autonomy. On this basis, any competent person should be allowed to make decisions that affect them and, therefore, a competent child should be given rights to self-determination: it is arbitrary and unfair to deny children rights because they are younger than adults. Alderson and Montgomery (1996), for example, emphasize that a child should have the right to give or withhold consent provided that he or she is considered competent by a doctor. This argument raises two extremely complex questions. First, how can competence be assessed? Second, is competence sufficient to entitle children and young people to full self-determination?

Children's competence

The new social studies of childhood has repeatedly attempted to reposition children as competent and rational (Mayall 2002, 2000), and as therefore deserving of the right to make autonomous decisions. Those who seek to defy conceptualizations of children as incompetent and irrational point to a literature within sociology that has attempted to show that children and young people are capable of producing coherent, rational, and competent accounts, are sensitive to issues of decision making and reflexive about their own involvement (for example Alderson 2000, 1993a; Hutchby and Moran-Ellis 1998b; Mayall 2002, 2000). Christensen (1998) advances the argument that competence is not a psychological property of an individual but a relational attribution that is socially constructed and negotiated. On this basis claims for the competence of children generally are made, and claims for children's incompetence based on psychological models are dismissed.

However, this position offers a simplistic analysis of how children's competence can be judged, and by denying psychology a place in contributing to understanding of children's competence, it risks producing a highly partisan and politically motivated view that is not grounded in relevant and appropriate empirical evidence and theory. In fact, much of the critique of psychology from the new social studies of childhood has referred to outdated and homogenized conceptions of developmental psychology and invoke, as we suggested in Chapter 1, something of a caricature. For example, the critique of the contributions of developmental psychology to investigating issues of competence have largely concentrated on Piagetian accounts of child development, and have not usually engaged with the range of different accounts of development and with more recent approaches to investigating children's abilities.

Within mainstream developmental psychology, the limitations of Piagetian conceptualizations of children's abilities and development have been recognized at least since the 1970s (for example McGarrigle and Donaldson 1974). In general terms, Piagetian accounts of children's development are believed to have understated the abilities of children, particularly preschool children, overemphasized differences in the abilities of younger children and older children (and even adults), and given insufficient recognition to the importance of contextual and domain specific factors in investigating individuals' abilities. Applications of Piagetian approaches to children's understanding of health and illness (for example, Brewster 1982; Perrin and Gerrity 1981) have also been criticized, both on methodological and conceptual grounds (Bird and Podmore 1990; Hergenrather and Rabinowitz 1991; Kalish 1996; Siegal and Peterson 1999). Specifically these have been criticized for inconsistencies in the criteria used for classifying children's reasoning about illness (Hergenrather and Rabinowitz 1991) and the assumption that children's concepts of illness are simpler and not just different to those of adults (Kalish 1996). Other researchers have suggested that Piagetian approaches to children's understanding of illness do not take sufficient account of the variation in children's experience, and the likelihood that children's concepts of illness reflect their limited experience and knowledge of illness (Bird and Podmore 1990; Crisp et al. 1996).

Newer approaches to cognitive development vary in the emphasis placed on general qualitative changes in how children reason and think as they develop, though most tend to reject the traditional Piagetian notion that cognitive development consists of stage-like transformations in content-independent logical structures (Goswami 2002b). Some suggest that younger children's reasoning abilities are not so different from those of older children, but what changes with development and experience is how children's knowledge is organized within particular subject or topic domains, and that development is more context-dependent and piecemeal than Piagetian models suggest. It is important to note that this allows for the possibility that with appropriate support, young children may be capable of understanding concepts previously thought to be beyond their reach. After investigating age-related differences in the organization of children's knowledge of illness, Hergenrather and Rabinowitz (1991) concluded that 6- to 7-year-olds had more accurate knowledge of illness causes, consequences and treatment than previous studies had suggested and that they can understand basics facts about disease processes. In an investigation of pre-school children's concepts of the causes and symptoms of illness, Kalish (1996) found little evidence to support the claims of Piagetian researchers that pre-school children's understanding of illness was limited to easily observable symptoms and that they believe all illnesses are contagious, while other work has suggested that 5-year-olds have some understanding of psychological states such as depression (Charman and Chandiramani 1995).

More generally, other research on child development has pointed to young children's understanding of mental, social, cultural and linguistic phenomena (Harris 1989; Siegal and Peterson 1996) and to their memory abilities (Peterson and Rideout 1998), all capacities that are likely to have some bearing on questions about children's competence. Research within developmental psychology has also pointed to wide-ranging individual differences in ability between children of the same age (Sternberg 2002).

While recognizing that the previous accounts of children's abilities may have underestimated children's abilities, developmental psychologists acknowledge limits to the cognitive and other competencies of young children. Kalish (1996) found that pre-schoolers' concepts of illness are less differentiated than those of adults. For example, they exhibit a greater tendency to assume that certain consequences or outcomes will apply to all illnesses. Hergenrather and Rabinowitz (1991) suggest that limitations in children's knowledge and differences in the cognitive organization of their knowledge can create problems for younger children in understanding about illness. In one of the few pieces of research to investigate cognitive processes in children with cancer, Chen et al. (2000) found that younger children showed less accurate recall of lumbar puncture procedures than older children. Other theorists point to the importance of considering developmental changes in information-processing speed, capacity and efficiency (Goswami 2002b), and in children's strategies for problem solving (Zelazo and Muller 2002). Peterson and Siegal (1999) note that accurate understanding of the causes and treatments for illness is only one of the elements involved in a child's cognitive competence to make medical decisions and point to the importance of being able to weigh probabilities and alternatives against one another. This requires an understanding of the long-term benefits and risks of the treatment proposed, as well as the immediate consequences.

Research within developmental psychology therefore suggests that young children have greater cognitive competencies than Piagetian researchers had previously anticipated.

> This view of young children as competent reasoners is very different to the more traditional notion that reasoning becomes increasingly logical with age. The traditional view was based on the false assumption that reasoning strategies are independent of context and content ... Now that more recent work in adult reasoning has shown that even supposedly efficient reasoners are affected by problem content and problem context, developmental views are gradually changing. Of course it would be absurd to suggest that there are no

developmental differences between children and adults or (between younger and older children). There are considerable differences in many experimental paradigms with age, but these differences may not be linked to the intrinsic logical requirements of the reasoning tasks instantiated in these paradigms. Rather they may reflect a variety of factors such as lack of knowledge about problem content, differences in basic mental capacities such as short term memory, ineffective general learning strategies such as use of appropriate mnemonic devices and metacognitive difficulties.

(Goswami 2002: 301)

What are children's views about participating in decision making?

Working within what James et al. (1998) would term the 'minority group' model of childhood, Alderson (1993a) interviewed 120 young people (aged 8–15 years) undergoing elective orthopaedic surgery for relief of chronic pain, disability or deformity. Most were veterans of surgery, having had on average five previous operations. A small proportion of young people wanted to be the 'main decider' (21 out of 120). Asked what they might do if they disagreed with their parents over the decision on surgery, more than a fifth (22 per cent) of boys and 11 per cent of girls said they would try to get their own way. This work also identified that many children were able to grasp the concepts of treatment and its consequences, and that 'I would like to see the age limits completely scrapped, and maturity brought in. As you grow up your age has a stereotype. I'm trying to escape from that stereotype' (Robin, aged 13, quoted in Alderson 1993a: 9).

Alderson and Montgomery (1996) draw the important conclusion that children who have experienced illness acquired competences and experiences that lead them to have greater maturity and insight in making decisions, a finding that is consistent with psychological research on the effect of experience of illness on the development of children's understanding of illness (Crisp et al. 1996).

If children can be competent, how can their competence be assessed?

The empirical literature importantly provides support for the position that many children, especially those who are veterans of illness, can produce coherent and rational views relevant to decisions about their care, and that some children would prefer to participate in such decisions. The literature can certainly be read as showing that there is no straightforward association between age and competence (Peterson and Siegal 1999), and that many children are capable of demonstrating mature and responsible capacity for decision making. In this sense, then, there is an alternative to the social construction of children as inherently incompetent and vulnerable and requiring protection. In some accounts, the finding that children and young people hold coherent views has taken the form of a challenge to the assumption that adults know the best interests of the child, and the argument that children should have rights *equal* to those of adults is made. However, there are several important caveats in attempting to apply the general findings of these studies to specific situations where decisions need to be made.

An obvious empirical point is that the literature in the new social studies of childhood is based on children who have agreed to take part in research studies, and may not be representative of all children and young people, particularly those confronted by life-threatening illness where decisions need to be made urgently and immediately with important consequences for children's survival, as is often the case in childhood cancer. Alderson's (1993a) study, for example, concerned children who were to have elective orthopaedic operations where the consequences of refusal of treatment were unlikely to be fatal, and where it was often possible to delay decisions to allow consideration of the issues and greater participation by the child.

Moroever, even the liberationists appear to accept that the right of self-determination requires that someone must have sufficient cognitive competence. The existing literature on children's competence cannot be read as meaning that all children are competent in all circumstances without reverting to notions of the 'universal child' so firmly rejected by the new social studies of childhood. The question then becomes one of how to determine whether *each individual child*, in *specific context*, is competent to make a *particular decision*. No satisfactory test of this exists (Ross 1997), though there are several proposals for how competence might be assessed. Alderson (1993a), for example, suggests that children should be able to understand the proposed treatment, be able to make a wise decision, and be free from coercion. Doig and Burgess (2000) attempt to specify what competence might involve (see Box 7.2). However, current proposals do not provide a clear, unambiguous, and objective means of assessing a particular child in a particular situation: a judgement still has to be made by somebody, presumably somebody attempting to act in the child's best interests.

Interestingly, the problems of finding a suitable way to determine competence has meant that even those working within a liberationist perspective, who most vociferously argue against age being used to determine qualification for decision making, end up falling back to some extent on notions of chronology as guiding assessment of competence. Some commentators have put the age at which children can competently reach a decision as 9 years (Roche 1999). Alderson and Montgomery (1996) propose, for a code of practice, that children of compulsory school age should be presumed to be competent, and the onus would lie on adults to demonstrate the child's

Box 7.2:   Competence in decision making

Being considered competent to make a decision implies:

- the ability to express the choice between alternatives;

- that the risks, benefits and alternatives are understood when various choices are considered;

- that rational and logical reasoning is demonstrated;

- that the choice is 'reasonable';

- that the choice is made without coercion.

(From Doig and Burgess 2000)

incompetence rather than requiring children to pass tests of competence which many adults might fail. They propose that capacity would be defined as being present when a child understands the type and purpose of the proposed treatment; in broad terms the nature and effects of the treatment; the principal benefits and risks; and the consequences of not receiving treatment. The code of practice would make it clear that a child's disagreement with a health professional could not be held as evidence of incompetence, and a child's refusal would be legally binding on health professionals. It is not clear how these judgements about children's understanding would be made in practice.

Is competence enough?

Those working within the liberationist paradigm would argue that disputes over decisions involving a young person's body should be resolved in favour of the child, as long as that young person can be judged to be competent. A fundamental problem concerns whether competence is a sufficient condition on which to prosecute a case for autonomy in decision making for children.

In childhood cancer, there are several important contexts to be considered in applying the principle that children and young people should have the authority to consent or refuse to medical attention and intervention. The extreme dependence of children on medical technology and tightly specified treatment protocols means that families and children are uniquely compromised in their choices and the extent to which they can exercise them if they wish to maximize their chances of survival. Moreover, as we have noted earlier, children with cancer have to suffer a great deal. They may become worn out, depressed and unwilling to endure any more, and this may affect their views about treatment aimed at longer-term outcomes. They may experience pain and fear that inhibit them in taking a long-term view. Those seeking to promote the long-term interests of children will want to take these issues into account alongside more general judgements of capacity and competence.

A key criticism of the demand that competence be the sole qualification for decision making is that it treats any attempt to overrule decisions by a competent child as illegitimate. It excludes adults, including parents, from making a decision that they believe better serves the child's interests. This position denies that adults (any adults) are capable of making a better informed, well-motivated decision than an individual child. It also creates a discourse of blame, in which an adult attempting to overrule a child is guilty of oppressive practice. It valorizes children as rational and competent, while simultaneously creating adults – all adults – as potential oppressors. Creating such a dichotomy between adults and children assumes all adults are on the same 'side' and neglects other axes of power and influence – for example, those that exist between adults, specifically between parents and professionals.

Indeed it is striking how little of the social science debate around children's rights has engaged with parents' rights, though an analysis of how the law operates (see earlier in this chapter) will show that parents can also be overruled by courts. An important literature has also shown the ways in which asymmetries of power in the medical consultation, expressed through ceremonial forms and etiquette rules can disadvantage parents in their attempts to engage in decision making relevant to their children in medical consultations (Gwyn 2002; Silverman 1987; Strong 1979). Other power relations may exist between other adult parties involved in decision making, and what Gabe et al. (2004) refer to as 'coalitions' may easily form, but these are not necessarily child versus adult – they may involve any combination of the child and the adult groupings. The assumption of an inherent hostility between child and adult is, therefore, likely to be flawed. Moreover, a simplistic characterization of adults as oppressive conceals the often agonized nature of negotiations between adults and children in attempts to secure children's well-being: 'But there were days when she wouldn't take [her medicines] and you're thinking oh God she's got to have them. And you're panicking and you're getting at her and she's getting upset. I think that was the most strenuous thing out of everything' (Mother of 10-year-old girl, quoted in Young et al. 2002: 1839).

In constituting children as individuals and privileging their rights to self-determination, the liberationist position fails to consider how granting children these rights might threaten the rights and emotional well-being of others, including those of parents and other carers. Decisions made by children with cancer will very often impose obligations on others or have consequences for them, including substantial emotional implications. To argue that young people be the sole decision makers neglects the rights of others who may be affected by the consequences of the decision, though we do recognize the limits to this argument.

Some of the problems with excluding the legitimacy of other perspectives from the decision-making process are illustrated by the case of Marco (Case study 3). His decision might be judged entirely competent and internally coherent, and as adequately reflecting his choices based on his priorities. His priority – to retain his leg – is indeed extremely important and rational on its own terms. However, a decision to refuse amputation is very likely to result in a long and very painful death. If the procedure were undertaken successfully, it is possible, and indeed likely, that his current priorities would be replaced by others as he adapts to his altered physical status (Albrecht and Devlieger 1999) and as he grows older, and his doctors and family would wish assume obligations to safeguard his ability to achieve these. Arguing that any attempt to do this represents oppressive practice simplifies a highly complex and sensitive set of negotiations and interactions.

Ross (1997) makes the unfashionable argument that even if children are competent, there is a morally significant difference between competent minors and adults. Though repeatedly emphasizing that children and adults share many points of similarity, her arguments are based on the *relative* differences between them, an observation that is strongly supported by much research within developmental psychology. She points out that one reason to limit children's present-day autonomy is to respect their lifetime autonomy. A second reason to limit the child's present-day autonomy is because children's decisions are based on limited world experience. Again, Ross points out that many adults also have limited world experience, but children have a *greater* potential for improving their knowledge base and for improving their skills of critical re-flection and self-control. Ross argues for family, rather than child, autonomy.

We would suggest that the liberationist tradition in relation to children's rights continues an attempt by those working within the new social studies of childhood to assign 'victimhood' to childhood. The process of assigning victim status serves not only a descriptive function, but also involves implicit instruction on how to view the victim, calls forward particular blame attri-butions and organizes 'proper' responses such as sympathy or righteous in-dignation (Holstein and Miller 1990). Taken together, the liberationist approach involves, therefore, a social construction of children and of their relationships with the adult world that may be no more legitimate than any other social construction.

The need to understand decision making in practice

As Gwyn et al. (2003) point out, the theoretical and practical aspects of in-creased participation in decision making have not been satisfactorily re-solved. Nowhere is this more true than for involvement in decision making by children with serious life-threatening diseases and their carers. Some of the early work on shared decision making in adults appeared to assume that all that was required to move towards more participative models was will and competence on the part of doctors. That this view is simplistic is now increasingly recognized. As Gwyn et al. (2003) note, practical issues are of considerable importance in understanding the extent to which shared decision making is possible: the bureaucratic problems of healthcare organisations and systems, the narrow temporal bandwidths, differential power and information gradients, and dissonance of explanatory models, all militate against equal participation in complex decisions. There are, moreover, important reasons to believe that some people may in fact prefer not to be 'decisive' when confronted by decisions about serious illness, and may experience the obligation to 'be free' as a burden. For example, patients' emotional needs in the context of severe or life-threatening illness may mean that they give little priority to shared decision making, and are more concerned about feeling cared for, by doctors in whom they can place their trust (Burkitt-Wright et al. 2004). Importantly, it has also been noted how, in constructing patients as agents in their own healthcare, models of shared decision making allow doctors to withdraw from responsibility from certain areas of patients' suffering and need (Salmon and Hall 2003).

Given the size and heat of the literature on children's participation in decision making, it is somewhat disturbing to discover the modest size and lack of sophistication of the empirical literature on decision making in childhood cancer. It is clear that much of the debate about has been preoccupied with consent, and been conducted within a bioethical discourse without the benefit of empirical foundations. A well-informed understanding of how decision making is handled in practice is noticeably absent, as has research that has elicited the perspectives of children with cancer and those that care for them, a proper recognition of the highly complex nature of decision making in relation to children, and evidence on the consequences of different approaches to decision making.

Research on involvement in decision making in childhood cancer

As we have noted earlier, the academic and political movement towards what has come to be known as 'patient partnership' has been gathering momentum for some time. A substantial body of empirical and theoretical work on adults is now beginning to emerge (Charles et al. 1999a; Gwyn et al. 2003). In the field of adult oncology, several studies have shown that patients generally have strong needs for information, but only a minority seek to assert control over decisions (Coulter 1997; Entwistle 2000). There has been much less research on issues of involvement in decision making in paediatrics, particularly in childhood cancer. Indeed a recent review was only able to cite a few references (Massimo 2004). Much of the research that has been conducted has been of poor quality, often relying on small surveys that are inconclusive and do little to illuminate process, or has focused solely on the issues of parental involvement in decision making. Much of the work also fails to attend to the complexities, for example failing to recognize the triadic nature of consultations and decision making. In particular, the child's role is rarely the focus of research (Tates and Meeuwesen 2001).

Some work has sought to identify children's and parents' preferences for involvement in decision making, though research on children's preferences is much more infrequent. Ellis and Leventhal (1993) report a survey of 50 children with cancer aged 8 to 17 years and their parents. Trust in the doctor was the most frequent reason for agreeing to treatment (90 per cent of children and 98 per cent of parents). Although most children wanted to be fully informed about their disease and its treatment, the majority of children (89 per cent) wanted the doctor to make treatment decisions, 7 per cent wanted their parents to make decisions, and 4 per cent wanted to make their own decisions. The majority of parents (69 per cent) in this study also wanted the doctor to decide, although almost a third (29 per cent) wanted to decide themselves and 2 per cent wanted their child to decide between treatment options.

Pyke-Grimm et al. (1999) conducted a survey of 58 parents of children in Canada, and reported that 52 per cent preferred a collaborative role, in which they shared responsibility for deciding treatment for the child; 29 per cent preferred a passive role, in which they left decisions to the clinicians; and 19 per cent preferred an active role, in which they made decisions having taken account of clinicians' opinions. A qualitative study used focus groups with 45 parents in the USA (Holm et al. 2003), described an advocacy role taken on by parents during treatment. This involved parents informing themselves about their child's medical status and needs, deciding about their child's medical treatment, limiting medical procedures, and actively and intentionally supporting and fostering relationships with medical staff. Parents described what appeared to be highly partnership-based models, where they were offered options by doctors and were able to select among them. They described working with medical staff to make decisions about scheduling treatment, including special events in their children's lives or their own work schedule. They also sought to limit specific treatment activities, for example, by refusing to wake children or intervening to improve communication with their child, or prevent incorrect treatment. A study on parents' decisions about complementary therapy use (Gagnon and Recklitis 2003) found that parents conceived of their role as very different from the role of an adult patient, and preferred active or collaborative forms of decision making. Tait et al.'s (2001) study, however, distinguished different preferences in relation to different decisions, and it is likely that future work will need to continue to make these distinctions (illustrated in our case studies), as well as exploring how it is that parents and children negotiate these decisions.

Issues of power are clearly hugely relevant to these negotiations, and are clearly an inescapable feature of child–adult relations, not one which can be eradicated by wishing it away. Moreover, Gabe et al. (2004) note recent work (for example Bendelow and Brady 2002) which is beginning to show that it would be quite wrong to suggest that children cannot and do not exercise their autonomy or 'countervailing power' in a variety of ways and for very different reasons. Children's social positioning is an active process as they continually monitor and evaluate their own behaviour, and, as Silverman (1987) points out, even those at the foothills of the mountains of power have strategic counters to play. As we noted earlier, 'coalitions' may be one manifestation of this.

The debates about adult power over those who belong to the social category of childhood become most acute, of course, when children and young wish to make choices which, in the judgement of others, may not serve their long-term welfare (see case studies). These debates are intensified during adolescence, when young people may be especially insistent on their right to self-determination. Research that has investigated children's views of the types of activities and practices that they believe should be under their own legitimate control has identified that issues such as choice of friends, appearance and leisure activities are felt by children to be within their own personal domain and should not be subject to interference by adults. Conflicts between children and their parents appear to become especially acute in adolescence, when young people often challenge their parents' definitions of personal domain and seek to assert their own control over a range of issues (Neff and Helwig 2002).

Brannen's (1996) important work on how the transition to adulthood is managed demonstrates that a variety of strategies is available to parents. They may select from among these to maintain control and fulfil their perceived obligations. For example, parents who draw upon a discourse of 'individual rights' and who emphasize the right of young people to create their own trajectory to adulthood might position themselves as 'friends' or 'confidantes' for their children, and may adopt more covert forms of control. Young people may use counter-strategies to fend off parents and create boundaries around their presumed autonomy, including withholding information. As we have shown in previous chapters, the public nature of childhood cancer and the positioning of the family and its constituent members in communication practices mean that neither covert control by parents nor withholding of information by children is likely to be possible. Power relations are thus brutally exposed, potentially creating extreme difficulties when the young person seeks to defend his or her autonomy, but those in authority seek to impose practices that appear most likely to secure the best clinical outcome. Attempts by young people to protect their identity as autonomous and independent in such situations may result in rejecting any advice from adults.

Seeking control may then come to be prioritized over making the 'best' decision, and in some circumstances young people may reject some options simply because an adult has recommended them.

It is clear that there are a number of different models that might be used in attempting to manage such situations, and the involvement of children in decision making more generally. O'Kane (2000), for example, describes the use of participatory approaches, using techniques such as a decision making charts and group activity days, used for exploring children's experiences of being looked after. However, the absence of research means that the consequences of even limited forms of participation in childhood cancer – for example inviting a child to have a say in a decision – are unknown. Some have suggested that participation is likely to be beneficial to children (for example, Peterson and Siegal 1999). However, in the absence of empirical evidence, it is difficult to be confident that asking the child to have a say and then making a decision that is inconsistent with their expressed wishes is in fact less damaging that simply informing the child of the decision and explaining the reasons for it; and it may be that the effects will be highly context-specific or dependent on precisely how negotiations are handled. It is also possible that more extended forms of decision making, where the child is given the right of veto or formal authority over the decision, could have even more unfortunate outcomes. For example, Alderson's (1993a) own work identified that responsibility for decision making is associated with the potential for blame and guilt: if something goes wrong, it is 'blamed' on the person who made the decision. The consequences of encouraging parents and children to make decisions which they may later come to regret, and which are more difficult to 'blame' on anyone else, require very careful assessment.

Conclusions

As Brannen and O'Brien (1996b) point out, any understanding of modern childhood in westernized societies must recognize the growth in the importance of parental *duties* and obligations, which has occurred at the same time as the diminishing of parental *rights* over children. They note that discourses of children's vulnerability and need for protection endure an uneasy coexistence with discourses about children's rights to empowerment, self-determination and participation. The status of children's status as decision makers are fiercely debated, with pragmatist approaches favouring participation by children in decisions with limited rights to consent or refuse to treatment, and those working in the liberationist tradition arguing that any competent child should be given full rights of consent.

As with our position on communication, we are not making an argument for or against children's involvement in decision making, but for evidence to inform the debates. Most of the debates have been conducted within a bioethical discourse without the benefit of empirical evidence, and some working within the new social studies of childhood have dismissed the contribution of developmental psychology. This degrading of psychology is unwarranted, and a proper scientific approach to understanding children's cognitive processes is essential to inform debates about competence, which are otherwise in danger of being driven by political imperatives rather than soundly based evidence. Though children's participation in decision making hinges on moral as well as empirical concerns, there are risks that the children's rights movement and the drive to seek and value users' views could result in adverse outcomes for children if untested models of partnership and user involvement are uncritically applied to childhood cancer (Dixon-Woods et al. 1999). Child partnership models need to be based on demonstration of the benefits of shared decision making, adequate investigation of the requirements for support, and evaluation of potential negative consequences.

8 Conclusions

In this chapter we conclude by reflecting briefly on the material we have presented and by identifying where the study of experiences of childhood cancer needs to go next. We began this book by arguing that a social science account of *living* with childhood cancer is needed. One important contribution of the 'new' social studies of childhood is to reposition children as agentic and reflexive. It will be clear from our discussions in this book that, whatever the weaknesses in the empirical base of social science study in this area, this is the appropriate way to conceptualize children and young people with cancer. Children and young people with cancer should be taken seriously as social agents in their own right, and be seen as active in giving meaning to their own experiences. They are also active participants in the emotional, biographical and physical work of having childhood cancer, including its strategic management.

We depart, however, from some of the other main tenets of the new social studies of childhood on a number of issues (recognizing that in this, we are taking the new social studies as a whole, and that there are different positions within it). We argue, first, that an interdisciplinary approach is needed, and that the dismissal or degrading of psychology has been misguided. We propose that the valorizing of children as rational and competent, and the associated characterization of adults as powerful oppressors, has potentially unfortunate implications for childhood cancer. Second, we argue that childhood cancer is not something that affects only children, and that the experiences of parents in particular need to be considered alongside those of children.

We conclude by noting that many of the issues we have raised in this book reflect the absence of a properly elaborated sociology of childhood illness to complement the psychology of childhood illness, and that much more thorough, rigorous and sophisticated empirical research and theorisation is required. An interpretive interdisciplinary approach is likely to offer the most fruitful way forward.

The need for an interdisciplinary approach

The new social studies of childhood has produced an almost entirely sociological account of childhood. It has, in much of its writing, explicitly taken on the role of 'reconstructing' childhood to debunk social constructions of children as inevitably incompetent and vulnerable, and of emphasizing children as 'being' rather than 'becoming'. Linked to this, there has been a push towards a politicization of childhood, often positioning occupants of the social category of childhood and occupants of the social category of adulthood in a minority/oppressor relationship, and arguing for an emancipatory agenda. In this, developmental psychology has been repeatedly attacked for presenting a linear picture of maturation and development that has been pervasive in its influence on medical and legal practice.

These positions are potentially problematic when applied to the question of how to understand experiences of childhood cancer. The clinical context, as we have emphasized throughout this book, is crucial. Children with cancer are, like anyone who is extremely ill with a life-threatening disease, very vulnerable; their vulnerability is not simply a social construction. This vulnerability is enhanced by their dependence on medical technologies, mostly using rigid protocols and lengthy periods of hospitalization, and involving many distressing symptoms and socially located disruptions, to secure their future well-being. To argue that children should be understood primarily as they are, rather than what they will become, risks reifying childhood generally, but for children with cancer it is an unhelpful and potentially damaging characterization, since their current suffering is so explicitly aimed towards their future survival. Their status as children further intensifies their vulnerability, but this is not simply or solely a social status; it is also a biological one. As we have shown throughout the book, the epidemiology of childhood cancer, and many of its effects and the effects of its treatment, are hugely variable according to the age of the child.

In these circumstances, the insistence that there must be 'open communication' with children, and that children should be involved in decisions about and able to consent or refuse medical treatments, has very serious implications. We stress the inappropriateness of adopting inflexible and rigid approaches to communication (whether in the direction of full disclosure or the reverse), particularly in the striking absence of research about the priorities and preferences of children in this sensitive and difficult area. As will be clear from our summary of the current evidence, preferences for information and involvement in decision making vary between children, but may also vary over time in the same child. The potential consequences of open communication and involvement in decision making are largely unknown, and there are many uncertainties about how disclosures of information and children's expressed views should be managed. How seriously the objection of a very ill child to being subject to a painful, frightening or distressing but necessary procedure should be taken into account needs to be considered within this very specific context. To argue that the often agonized efforts of parents and staff to gain children's cooperation are simply the actions of an oppressive majority is to risk offering a crude and simplistic account of a highly complex situation.

Similarly, to argue that information is withheld from children through taking advantage of an unequal balance of power coupled with the paternalistic instincts of adults does not do full justice to the complexities of situations in childhood cancer and the positioning of the parties involved. For example, there is a need to recognize the ways in which children are strategic in their use of silence in consultations, and in their use of parents as envoys and communication buffers. We propose that imposing certain forms of uniform 'rights' on children in relation to information and decision making is in fact potentially oppressive (effectively functioning as a prior determination of their best interests). Much more needs to be done to explore the extent to which (individual) children really wish to be decisive and the long-term outcomes of those decisions, their preferences regarding the form of their relationships with professionals, and how their needs, including emotional and informational needs, can be better met. In this, there is a need to be clear that some issues are not easily tractable; once the explanation that it is not simply lack of will that holds adults back from sharing information and decisions with children falls away, other explanations demand far more complex and demanding solutions.

These issues also highlight the need for theorizing of childhood illness to take account of the science of development, to avoid, for example, confounding the general social competence of children with specific competences in medical decision making. Here, the damaging consequences of the caricaturing of developmental psychology that appears throughout the new social studies of childhood is most evident. As we have shown, developmental psychology is much more sophisticated and diverse than its critics have given it credit for, and has a vital role to play in informing not only debates about the characteristic cognitive processes of children at different ages, but also in the assessment of individual competences.

Study of these important aspects of childhood cancer is likely to involve approaches that integrate contributions from sociology and psychology, and that use methods including ethnography and conversation analysis as well as directly accessing the views of children and their families. The role of health professionals other than doctors will be a key interest of this future work.

The family and childhood cancer

Throughout this book we have argued that families also have experiences of childhood cancer that are just as deserving of study as those of children. To separate out experiences of families and children is to engage in a form of reification that conceals dynamic and interdependent processes and negotiations. The experiences of parents are especially important and interesting, though attention also needs to be given to siblings and other socially adjacent people. Lupton and Barclay (1997) describe how parents have acquired a whole series of obligations in relation to their children, particularly in relation to their health and welfare. Childhood cancer serves as a particular form of the intensification of parenthood. Parenting a child with cancer needs to be recharacterized to draw attention to how parents' identities and social obligations position them in relation to the medical world, to highlight the emotional work carried by parents, and to show how becoming, and being, a parent of a child with cancer invites surveillance of parenthood. We are conscious, of course, that most research has focused on accounts of mothers, and that there is risk that research could (unwittingly) reinforce aspects of motherhood as 'natural' and non-negotiable, rather than reflexively produced in response to dominant social and discursive constructions. Clearly, the ways in which family members come to recognize and adopt norms and roles in relation to childhood cancer will be an important aspect of future research. So too will be exploration of different forms of families, including children who are in the care of social services, whose parents are unable or unwilling to accept the roles that are socially prescribed for them.

The need for research

We have identified many weaknesses in the evidence base of experiences of childhood cancer. Where we have been most critical of psychology in this book has, of course, been in relation to its preoccupation with psychological morbidity. We acknowledge that identifying psychological outcomes of childhood cancer is important, but the dominance of this approach has been unfortunate. Moreover, some of the research on the psychosocial aspects of childhood cancer has been of poor quality, and has often produced wildly conflicting findings that do little to provide enlightenment, or been so inconclusive as to be uninformative. The future should see fewer studies with uncontrolled designs, conducted using small sample sizes from single centres, and lacking in statistical power.

We would urge that, drawing on traditions within sociology and psychology, interpretive perspectives and methods consistent with these are needed to fully engage with the notion that children are active participants in the social construction of both their experiences and their illness. They are also active in the interpretive reproduction of cultures around their illness (on children's wards, for example). However, qualitative work in the area of childhood cancer has also been disappointing, both in quantity and, very often, in quality. Some of it of limited value, offering little beyond description, is based on inappropriate samples, and lacks insight or explanatory value. The future should see much better-designed studies that attempt much more sophisticated forms of theorization.

Many questions need to be addressed in the social science study of experiences of childhood cancer, many of which we have highlighted throughout the book. We will draw attention to a few important further issues. First, we have noted that a properly elaborated sociology of childhood illness is absent. This poses major challenges for those attempting to theorize in a specific area such as childhood cancer. There is an urgent need to begin to distinguish the ways that a sociology of childhood illness might draw on constructs already developed within the sociology of adult chronic illness, and to identify where completely new forms of theorizing are required. As we have shown, there is some evidence that many existing constructs have considerable explanatory value as far as experiences of chronic childhood illness is concerned, but much more needs to be done to explore and develop them. In taking the specific field of childhood cancer forward, it is clear that there is a particular need to attend to the different sub-groups. Different forms of tumours may have very different effects, and there is a real need establish the extent to which they should be seen as different diseases. Much more, too, needs to be done to understand the experiences of children of different ages.

The absence of gender from research and theory on childhood cancer thus far is very striking. There is, for example, almost no research on the gendered experience of childhood cancer, but research in other areas of childhood illness demonstrates that this may well be an important feature. Williams (2002), for example, identifies that illness constitutes a threat to masculine identity, and that boys are more likely to aim to pass as normal and healthy, whereas girls may be more likely to confide in friends. These gendered aspects of the disruptive effects of illness may have very different consequences for the ways in which parents are implicated; mothers and sons may engage in a silent conspiracy to promote a fiction of health and independence, while daughters may have more autonomy, but less support. To what extent these insights apply to childhood cancer is unknown. Little is known either about the gendering of caring for childhood cancer itself. Williams (2002) identified that mothers help their adolescent sons in ways that are invisible to them, prompted by gendered social expectations of appropriate disease management. The study of fathers has been notably lacking, though whether this reflects fathers' more minor (or different) care-giving roles in families of a child with cancer, or a focus of research, or limitations of the research process that are themselves founded on social constructions (for example, of mothers as spokespersons for the family, the natural candidates to offer narratives) is unclear.

Although we acknowledged that we were focused on experiences of cancer within westernized societies, there are intriguing hints in the literature of sociocultural differences that would benefit from cross-cultural and cross-national research. For example a body of evidence suggests that in China and Taiwan, very different belief systems may exist about the causation and appropriate treatment of childhood cancer. This may result distinctive attitudes towards biomedicine, including increased use of alternative therapies (sometimes completely substituting for conventional biomedicine) and patterns of 'drop out' from conventional treatment that are not typically seen in westernized countries. Yeh et al. (1999) for example, in a study of Taiwanese parents whose children dropped out of treatment for childhood cancer, describes parents' search for religious explanations and the use of fortune tellers, and reported extremely poor communication with medical professionals.

The need for the development of interpretive approaches in the field of late effects is very evident. The lack of sophistication of the field is especially disappointing because late effects represent a particularly interesting area in which to develop theory: late effects represent symptoms and outcomes that appear or persist after the illness has been 'cured', but they also represent the long-term narrative and biographical effects of a disease in childhood. Conceptually, they form a discontinuity with the study of chronic illness by their appearance after 'cure', and they demonstrate the fallacy evident in the new social studies of childhood of an insistent focus on childhood as 'being' rather than 'becoming'.

Much more work needs to be done on services and on how these can best be organized to meet the needs and priorities of children and their families. Already there is evidence of the important role that appropriate services play in the well-being of young people with cancer (Haase and Phillips 2004), but this is an area ripe for development. Finally, an agenda about people's experiences of participating in research about childhood cancer would address many important questions and help in the development of methodologies that are grounded in the priorities and preferences of participants.

Methods for moving forward with research

In considering how research might move forward, it is clear that much hinges on the development of appropriate methods for accessing, analysing and representing the views of children and others who share in the experience of childhood cancer. Debates about the ways in which children and childhood should be researched highlight the fractures in the contemporary social science of childhood. The attempt within the new social studies to reposition children as deserving of attention in their own right, very often linked to a political agenda about the emancipation of children, has resulted in a call for the use of research in order to allow the authentic voices of children to be heard: 'The task of the social scientist is to work for the right of people to have a voice and be heard. In the case of children, ''age'', is perhaps one of the most dominant factors used to discriminate against children being heard and listened to' (Christensen and Prout 2002: 483). However, there is an unresolved methodological debate about how children should be researched, and in particular a debate about whether 'special' techniques are required to study children.

Debates about methodologies for researching children

Some authors (for example, Greig and Taylor 1999) emphasize the 'special-ness' of children and the need for specific research techniques to allow re-search with children, describing a range of techniques including drawing, playing (for example, using dolls and puppets), and story completion. Others working within the new social studies of childhood, particularly within the 'minority group' model, argue that using 'special' techniques risk reinforcing the notion of children as 'other' (James et al. 1998). A strong argument is made in particular against assuming that methodologies must be based on the age of children.

> (Thus) we might well expect to see patterns of difference in social behaviour between one age group and another; the danger lies in assuming that these social differences are the inevitable or even ne-cessary outcome of children's age or biological development . . . And yet so seductive is this framing, so familiar are we with models of child development, that many research designs uncritically in-corporate some aspects of an age-based methodology as if it were a 'natural' and irrevocable part of childhood.
>
> (James et al. 1998: 174)

Taking up these themes, Oakley (1994: 27) argues that: 'Most supposed differences between children and adults as research subjects disappear on closer inspection.' The major issues of the researcher–researched relationship are thus argued to be essentially the same with children as they are with adults (Brannen et al. 1994). These issues include the power relations of the researcher and the researcher, the need to explain fully the research, the need to attend to disparities between the class, ethnicity and gender of researchers and researcher, and the need to handle sensitive topics appropriately. Harden et al. (2000), for example, make the case that the use of 'special' methods is unnecessary, and that children can be engaged in research through conven-tional techniques, such as conversational interviews, already used with adults, although they do recognize a role for using play-based activities to prompt discussion. Christensen and James (2000) argue similarly that when choosing methods for working with children the basic principle is as it would be with any other piece of research (with adults): the methods must suit the people involved in the study, the kinds of research questions being investigated, and the specific social and cultural context of the research.

However, there are contradictions even within this position. While arguing on the one hand that 'special' methods are not needed, the need for a democratization, to provide opportunities for children to resist the researchers' control of the research process, has been emphasized (Mayall 1994a). This has often taken the form of arguing for the involvement of children themselves in the research process, encouraging them to collect data and assist in its analysis, and drawing on a comparison with feminist research, where it is proposed that research about women is far more insightful if it uses women researchers (Alderson 2001). This model of using age-adjacent researchers would seem to qualify as a 'special' technique, since it is not used with adults. There are few examples as yet of this model in childhood cancer research, but it is likely to require more critical evaluation than it has yet received. For example the ethics and issues that arise in asking children to collect data (or even analyse data) from other, very ill children would need careful assessment.

There are other problems with approaches that seek to downplay the significance of age as an important consideration in research design. James et al. (1998) may, as we pointed out earlier, describe age-based methodologies as seductive rather than sound, but it may well be that they are necessary: there are stubborn realities about what children are characteristically like at particular ages (4-year-olds, for example, are characteristically *not like* 8-year-olds) that may need to be designed into studies. Similarly, the argument that children are competent is repeatedly asserted rather than demonstrated in this literature, but, as we have already argued, such a claim might not survive a reading of contemporary developmental psychology.

Children's narratives

In this respect the lack of research about social science methods for investigating children and childhood is very notable, but clearly requires exploration. An example arises in relation to narrative interviews. For sociologists, the narrative interview has, of course, provided researchers with very rich and potent insights into adults' experiences of chronic illness, including cancer. It is important that we begin to investigate whether children's narratives are fundamentally different in both form and function from those of adults; to explore whether the form of children's narratives varies according to developmental age and 'illness' age, and to analyse the extent to which their narratives follow 'adult' conventions and whether they incorporate distinctive elements of fantasy, myth or received knowledge. It will be particularly important to look at 'ownership' of narratives: children may feel that their story is owned by others, perhaps particularly by their parents. Similarly, the functions that children perform in telling their stories require study: for children, some of that function, at least, may simply be the telling and the holding of someone's attention. Clearly, both theoretical and empirical research is needed into children's narratives.

Other methodological concerns

Similarly, although frequently advocated by those working within the new social studies of childhood, focus groups raise important ethical, and other, challenges in research with families of a child with cancer. Practical issues represent a serious barrier to organizing focus groups, which require people to be in the same place at the same time. For families of a child with cancer, making arrangements of this type may be extremely difficult, and may discourage certain types of families from participating. Other issues arise in relation to known problems in focus groups, including the risk of loss of confidentiality, because focus group participants may not feel bound by the same ethics as the researchers. People may offer confidences in focus groups which they later regret having shared publicly, while others may feel uncomfortable and silenced by dominant characters in the group. Peer expectations may arise in the group and produce apparent consensus while excluding dissonant views. Some participants can become bored or excluded by others, and the perception of the adult as an authority is difficult to manage (Goodenough et al. 2003). Overall, focus groups require careful handling, especially when they involve sensitive issues such as childhood cancer.

It will also be important to recognize that in many cases accounts from children will not provide complete insight into their experiences. In Chapter 2, for example, we showed that parents function as chroniclers and witnesses of their children's experiences of obtaining a diagnosis of childhood cancer. Parents' roles in offering accounts about their children should be acknowledged and valued, though clearly the methodological issues about interpreting accounts from third parties are paramount in the appropriate use of such material. Parents' narratives about themselves, of course, will continue to provide important insights into their own experiences.

Ethnography is clearly a hugely promising methodology for studying experiences of childhood cancer, but more research and reflexive accounts about conducting ethnography in this area are needed. Harden et al. (2000) note some of the difficulties associated with mounting ethnographic studies of children, however. They point, for example, to problems of access, particularly to sites involving family life. Hospitals may be relatively easy places to access; the frequent presence of an observer in the home may be much less acceptable, but may be where much of the action takes place. Shaw (1996) and Mauthner (1997) discusses the problems of trust that arise in conducting research using qualitative techniques with children. Ethnographic work raises particular problems, because of the potential for children (and parents) to develop trusting relationships with researchers. Such relationships may subsequently cause discomfort when research findings result in participants feeling that they have been betrayed by a friend. Disclosures, or allegations of physical, emotional or sexual harm may be made, which may require researchers to break confidentiality and intervene. Ethnographers may witness unacceptable or risky behaviour, and experience acute dilemmas about whether and when to intervene.

It will also be important to explore issues that impact upon the experiences of childhood cancer but which cannot be directly accessed solely by research with children or parents themselves. An understanding of the social construction of childhood cancer, for example, is essential in explaining the experiences of families of a child with cancer. Work on the media construction of childhood cancer, and further investigation into lay views of childhood cancer, is now needed.

Conclusions

An important reason for re-examining childhood cancer in the way we have done in this book concerns the opportunities it would offer to the social science study of childhood and childhood illness generally. Rethinking childhood cancer must involve a recognition of the contribution of the social sciences conceived broadly, and an interdisciplinary, interpretive perspective on how experiences of childhood cancer can be understood and studied. Such a project must include, above all, an emphasis on how those affected by childhood cancer – children themselves as well as their families – understand and give meaning to their experiences.

Bibliography

Alanen, L. (2001) Explorations in generational analysis, in Alanen, L. and Mayall, B., *Conceptualizing Child–Adult Relations*. London: RoutledgeFalmer.

Alanen, L. and Mayall, B. (2001) *Conceptualizing Child–Adult Relations*. London: RoutledgeFalmer.

Albrecht, G. and Devlieger, P. (1999) The disability paradox: high quality of life against all the odds. *Social Science and Medicine* 48, 977–88.

Albritton, K. and Bleyer, W. (2003) The management of cancer in the older adolescent. *European Journal of Cancer* 39, 2584–99.

Alderson, P. (1993a) *Children's Consent to Surgery*. Buckinghamshire: Open University Press.

Alderson, P. (1993b) European charter of children's rights. *Bulletin of Medical Ethics* 13–15.

Alderson, P. (1994) Researching children's rights to integrity, in Mayall, B. *Children's Childhoods Observed and Experienced*. London: Falmer.

Alderson, P. (2000) *Young People's Rights: Exploring Beliefs, Principles and Practice*. London: Save the Children/Jessica Kingsley.

Alderson, P. (2001) Research by children. *International Journal of Social Research Methodology* 4, 139–53.

Alderson, P. and Montgomery, J. (1996) *Health Care Choices: Making Decisions with Children*. London: Institute for Public Policy Research.

Allen, R., Newman, S. and Souhami, R. (1997) Anxiety and depression in adolescent cancer: findings in patients and parents. *European Journal of Cancer* 33, 1250–5.

American Academy of Pediatrics (1995) Informed consent, parental permission, and assent in pediatric practice. *Pediatrics* 95, 314–17.

Anholt, U., Fritz, G. and Keener, M. (1993) Self-concept in survivors of childhood and adolescent cancer. *Journal of Psychosocial Oncology* 11, 1–16.

Annequin, D., Tourniaire, B. and Massiou, H. (2000) Migraine and headache in childhood and adolescence. *Pediatric Clinics of North America* 47, 617–31.

Archard, D. (1993) *Children, Rights and Childhood*. London: Routledge.

Archard, D. and Macleod, C. (2002) Introduction, in Archard, D. and Macleod, C. M., *The Moral and Political Status of Children*. Oxford, Oxford University Press.

Aries, P. (1962) *Centuries of Childhood: A Social History of Family Life*. London: Cape.

Arksey, H. and Sloper, P. (1999) Disputed diagnoses: the cases of RSI and childhood cancer. *Social Science and Medicine* 49, 483–97.

Armstrong, D. (2003) *An Outline of Sociology as Applied to Medicine*. Oxford: Oxford University Press.

Atkin, K. and Ahmad, W. (2000) Family care-giving and chronic illness: how parents cope with a child with sickle cell disorder or thalassaemia. *Health and Social Care in the Community* 8, 57–69.

Barakat, L., Kazak, A., Gallagher, P., Meeske, K. and Stuber, M. (2000) Posttraumatic stress symptoms and stressful life events predict the long-term adjustment of survivors of childhood cancer and their mothers. *Journal of Clinical Psychology in Medical Settings* 7, 189–96.

Barakat, L., Kazak, A. and Meadows, A. (1997) Families surviving childhood cancer: a comparison of posttraumatic stress symptoms with families of healthy children. *Journal of Pediatric Psychology* 22, 843–59.

Barr, R. (2001) The adolescent with cancer. *European Journal of Cancer* 37, 1523–7.

Barrera, M., Chung, J., Greenberg, M. and others (2002) Preliminary investigation of a group intervention for siblings of pediatric cancer patients. *Children's Health Care* 31, 13.

Baruch, G. (1981) Moral tales: parents' stories of encounters with the health professions. *Sociology of Health and Illness* 3, 273–95.

Bauman, L., Drotar, D., Leventhal, J. and others (1997) A review of psychosocial interventions for children with chronic health conditions. *Pediatrics* 100, 244–51.

Bendelow, G. and Brady, G. (2002) Experiences of ADHD: children, health research and emotion work, in Bendelow, G., Carpenter, M., Vautier, C. and Williams, S., *Gender, Health and Healing: the Public/Private Divide*. London: Routledge.

Benporath, S. (2003) Autonomy and vulnerability: on just relations between adults and children. *Journal of Philosophy of Education* 37, 127–45.

Beresford, B. and Sloper, P. (2003) Chronically ill adolescents' experiences of communicating with doctors: a qualitative study. *Journal of Adolescent Health* 33, 172–9.

Bird, J. and Podmore, V. (1990) Children's understandings of health and illness. *Psychology and Health* 4, 175–85.

Bithell, J., Dutton, S., Draper, G. and Neary, N. (1994) Distribution of childhood leukaemias and non-Hodgkin's lymphomas near nuclear installations in England and Wales. *BMJ* 309, 501–5.

Blacklay, A., Eiser, C., Ellis, A. and others (1998) The development and evaluation of an information booklet for adult survivors of cancer in childhood. *Archives of Disease in Childhood* 78, 340–4.

Bleyer, W. (2002) Cancer in older adolescents and young adults: epidemiology, diagnosis, treatment, survival, and importance of clinical trials. *Medical and Pediatric Oncology* 38, 1–10.

Bluebond-Langner, M. (1974) I know do you? Awareness and communication in terminally ill children, in Schoenburg, B., Carr, A., Peretz, D., and Kutscher, A., *Anticipatory Grief*. New York: Columbia.

Bluebond-Langner, M. (1978) *The Private Worlds of Dying Children*. Princeton: Princeton University Press.

Bluebond-Langner, M. (1996) *In the Shadow of Illness: Parents and Siblings of the Chronically Sick Child*. Princeton: Princeton University Press.

Bluebond-Langner, M., Perkel, D. and Goertzel, T. (1991) The impact of an oncology camp experience. *Journal of Psychosocial Oncology* 9, 67–80.

BMA (2001) *Consent, Rights and Choices in Healthcare for Children and Young People*. London: BMJ Books.

Bourdieu, P. (1990) *In Other Words: Essays Towards a Reflexive Sociology*. London: Routledge.

Brannen, J. (1996) Discourses of adolescence: young people's independence and autonomy within families, in Brannen, J. and O'Brien, M., *Children in Families: Research and Policy*. London: Falmer Press.

Brannen, J., Dodd, K., Oakley, A. and Storey, P. (1994) *Young People, Health and Family Life*. Buckingham: Open University Press.

Brannen, J. and O'Brien, M. (1995) Childhood and the sociological gaze: paradigms and paradoxes. *Sociology* 29, 729–39.

Brannen, J. and O'Brien, M. (1996a) *Children in Families: Research and Policy*. Hampshire: Falmer Press.

Brannen, J. and O'Brien, M. (1996b) Introduction, in Brannen, J. and O'Brien, M., *Children and Families: Research and Policy*. London: Falmer Press.

Brazier, M. (2003) *Medicine, Patients and the Law*. London: Penguin.

Brewster, A. (1982) Chronically ill hospitalised children's concepts of their illness. *Pediatrics* 69, 355–62.

Brighouse, H. (2002) What rights (if any) do children have? in Archard, D. and Macleod, C. M., *The Moral and Political Status of Children*. Oxford: Oxford University Press.

Brown, K. and Barbarin, O. (1996) Gender differences in parenting a child with cancer. *Social Work in Health Care* 22, 53–71.

Brown, R., Kaslow, N., Hazzard, A. and others (1992) Psychiatric and family functioning in children with leukaemia and their parents. *Journal of the American Academy of Child and Adolescent Psychiatry* 31, 495–502.

Burkitt-Wright, E., Holcombe, C. and Salmon, P. (2004) Doctor's communication of trust, care and respect in breast cancer: qualitative study. *British Medical Journal* 328, 864.

Burman, E. (1994) *Deconstucting Developmental Psychology*. London: Routledge.

Bury, M. (1982) Chronic illness as biographical disruption. *Sociology of Health and Illness* 4, 167.

Bury, M. (1986) Social constructionism and the development of medical sociology. *Sociology of Health and Illness* 5, 1–24.

Bury, M. (2001) Illness narratives: fact or fiction? *Sociology of Health and Illness* 23, 263–85.

Butler, I. (1996) Children and the sociology of childhood, in Butler, I. and Shaw, I.

A Case of Neglect? Children's Experiences and the Sociology of Childhood. Aldershot, Avebury.

Byrne, A., Morton, J. and Salmon, P. (2001) Defending against children's pain: a qualitative analysis of nurses' responses to children's postoperative pain. *Journal of Psychosomatic Research* 50, 69–76.

Byrne, J., Fears, T., Steinhorn, S. and others (1989) Marriage and divorce after childhood and adolescent cancer. *Journal of the American Medical Association* 262, 2693–9.

Cabral, D. and Tucker, L. (1999) Malignancies in children who initially present with rheumatic complaints. *Journal of Pediatrics* 134, 53–7.

Callery, P. (1997) Paying to participate: financial, social and personal costs to parents of involvement in their children's care in hospital. *Journal of Advanced Nursing* 35, 746–52.

Carey, S. (1985) *Conceptual Change in Childhood.* Cambridge, MA: MIT Press.

Charles, C., Gafni, A. and Whelan, T. (1999a) Decision-making in the physician-patient encounter: revisiting the shared treatment decision-making model. *Social Science and Medicine* 49, 651–61.

Charles, C., Whelan, T. and Gafni, A. (1999b) What do we mean by partnership in making decisions about treatment? *BMJ* 319, 780–2.

Charman, T. and Chandiramani, S. (1995) Children's understanding of physical illnesses and psychological states. *Psychology and Health* 10, 145–53.

Chen, E., Zeltzer, L., Craske, M. and others (2000) Children's memories for painful cancer treatment procedures: implications for distress. *Child Development* 71, 933–47.

Chesler, M. and Parry, C. (2001) Gender roles and/or styles in crisis: an integrative analysis of the experience of fathers of children with cancer. *Qualitative Health Research* 11, 363–83.

Chesler, M., Paris, J. and Barbarin, O. A. (1986) 'Telling' the child with cancer: parental choices to share information with ill children. *Journal of Pediatric Psychology* 11, 497–516.

Christensen, P. (2000) Childhood and cultural constitution of vulnerable bodies, in Prout, A., *The Body, Childhood and the Society.* London: Macmillan.

Christensen, P. (2004) The health-promoting family: a conceptual framework for future research. *Social Science and Medicine* 59, 377–87.

Christensen, P. and James, A. (2000) *Research with Children: Perspectives and Practices.* London: RoutledgeFalmer.

Christensen, P. and Prout, A. (2002) Working with ethical symmetry in social research with children. *Childhood* 9, 477–97.

Christensen, P. (1998) Difference and similarity: how children's competence is constituted in illness and its treatment, in Hutchby, I. and Moran-Ellis, J., *Children and Social Competence: Arenas of Action.* London: Falmer.

Claflin, C. and Barbarin, O. (1991) Does 'telling' less protect more? Relationships among age, information disclosure, and what children with cancer see and feel. *Journal of Pediatric Psychology* 16, 169–91.

Clarke, J. and Fletcher, P. (2003) Communication issues faced by parents who have a child diagnosed with cancer. *Journal of Paediatric Oncology Nursing* 20, 175–91.

Clarke, S., Davies, H., Jenney, M., Glaser, A. and Eiser, C. (in press) Parental communication and children's behaviour following diagnosis of childhood leukaemia. *Psycho-Oncology*.

Clarke-Steffen, L. (1993a) A model of the family transition to living with childhood cancer. *Cancer Practice* 1, 285–92.

Clarke-Steffen, L. (1993b) Waiting and not knowing: the diagnosis of cancer in a child. *Journal of Pediatric Oncology Nursing* 10, 146–53.

Clarke-Steffen, L. (1997) Reconstructing reality: family strategies for managing childhood cancer. *Journal of Pediatric Nursing* 12, 278–87.

Coffey, A. and Atkinson, P. (1996) *Making Sense of Qualitative Data*. Thousand Oaks, CA: Sage.

Cohen, D., Friedrich, W., Jaworski, T., Copeland, D. and Pendergrass, T. (1994) Pediatric cancer: predicting sibling adjustment. *Journal of Clinical Psychology* 50, 303–19.

Cohn, R., Goodenough, B., Foreman, T. and Suneson, J. (2003) Hidden financial costs in treatment for childhood cancer: an Australian study of lifestyle implications for families absorbing out-of-pocket expenses. *Journal of Pediatric Hematology and Oncology* 25, 854–63.

Collins, J., Byrnes, M., Dunkel, I., Lapin, J., Nadel, T., Thaler, H., Polyak, T., Rapkin, B. and Portenoy, R. (2000) The measurement of symptoms in children with cancer. *Journal of Pain and Symptom Management* 19, 363–77.

Collins, J., Devine, T., Dick, G., Johnson, E., Kilham, H., Pinkerton, C., Stevens, M. T. H. and Portenoy, R. (2002) The measurement of symptoms in young children with cancer: the validation of the memorial symptom assessment scale in children aged 7–12. *Journal of Pain and Symptom Management* 23, 10–16.

Comaroff, J. and Maguire, P. (1981) Ambiguity and the search for meaning: childhood leukaemia in the modern clinical context. *Social Science and Medicine* 15B, 115–23.

Corsaro, W. (1997) *The Sociology of Childhood*. London: Pine Forge Press.

Cotterill, S., Parker, L., Malcolm, A., Reid, M., More, L. and Craft, A. (2000) Incidence and survival for cancer in children and young adults in the North of England 1968–1995: a report from the northern region young persons' malignant disease registry. *British Journal Of Cancer* 83, 397–403.

Coulter, A. (1997) Partnership with patient: the pros and cons of shared decision making. *Journal of Health Services Research and Policy* 35, 276–81.

Crisp, J., Ungerer, J. and Goodnow, J. (1996) The impact of experience on children's understanding of illness. *Journal of Pediatric Psychology* 21, 57–72.

Cummins, C., Winter, H., Maric, R., Cheng, K., Silcocks, P., Varghese, C. and Batlle, G. (2001) Childhood cancer in the south Asian population of England (1990–1992). *British Journal of Cancer* 84, 1215–8.

Cuttini, M., Da Fre, M., Haupt, R., Deb, G., Baronci, C. and Tamaro, P. (2003) Survivors of childhood cancer: using siblings as a control group (letter). *Pediatrics* 112, 1454–5.

Davies, B., Whitsett, S., Bruce, A. and McCarthy, P. (2002) A typology of fatigue in children with cancer. *Journal of Pediatric Oncology Nursing* 19, 12–21.

Davis, F. (1963) *Passage Through Crisis*. Indianapolis, IN: Bobbs-Merrill.

De Inocencio, J. (2004) Epidemiology of musculoskeletal pain in primary care. *Archives of Disease in Childhood* 89, 431–4.

Denzin, N. (1977) *Childhood Socialization*. San Francisco, CA: Jossey Bass.

Department of Health (2000) *Referral Guidelines for Suspected Cancer* London: Department of Health.

Dingwall, R. (1994) Litigation and the threat to medicine, in Gabe, J., Kelleher, D. and Williams, G., *Challenging Medicine*. London: Routledge.

Dixon-Woods, M. (2001) Writing wrongs? An analysis of published discourses about the use of patient information leaflets. *Social Science and Medicine* 52, 1417–32.

Dixon-Woods, M., Findlay, M., Young, B., Cox, H. and Heney, D. (2001) Parents' accounts of obtaining a diagnosis of childhood cancer. *Lancet* 357, 670–4.

Dixon-Woods, M., Seale, C., Young, B., Findlay, M. and Heney, D. (2003) Representing childhood cancer: accounts from newspapers and parents. *Sociology of Health and Illness* 25, 143–64.

Dixon-Woods, M., Young, B. and Heney, D. (1999) Partnerships with children. *BMJ* 319, 778–80.

Dobrovoljac, M., Hengartner, H., Boltshauser, E. and Grotzer, M. (2002) Delay in the diagnosis of paediatric brain tumours. *European Journal of Pediatrics* 161, 663–7.

Docherty, S. (2003) Symptom experiences of children and adolescents with cancer. *Annual Review of Nursing Research* 21, 123–49.

Dockerty, J., Draper, G., Vincent, T., Rowan, S. and Bunch, K. (2001) Case-control study of parental age, parity and socio-economic level in relation to childhood cancers. *International Journal of Epidemiology* 30, 1428–37.

Dockerty, J., Skegg, D. and Williams, S. (2003) Economic effects of childhood cancer on families. *Journal of Paediatric Child Health* 39, 254–8.

Dockerty, J., Wilkins, S. and McGee, R. (2000) Impact of childhood cancer on the mental health of parents. *Medical and Pediatric Oncology* 35, 475–83.

Doig, C. and Burgess, E. (2000) Withholding life-sustaining treatment: are adolescents competent to make these decisions? *CMAJ* 162, 1585–8.

Dolgin, M., Blumensohn, R., Mulhern, R., Sahler, O., Roghmann, Carpenter, P., Sargent, J., Barbarin, O., Copeland, D. and Zeltzer, L. (1997) Sibling adaptation to childhood cancer collaborative study: cross-cultural aspects. *Journal of Psychosocial Oncology* 15, 1–14.

Downie, A. (1999) Consent to medical treatment whose view of welfare? *Family Law* 29, 818–21.

Dreifaldt, A., Carlberg, M. and Hardell, L. (2004) Increasing incidence rates of childhood malignant diseases in Sweden during the period 1960–1998. *European Journal of Cancer* 40, 1351–60.

Drew, S. (2003) Self reconstruction and biographical revisioning: survival following cancer in childhood and adolescence. *Health* 7, 181–99.

Eden, O., Black, I., MacKinlay, G. and Emery, A. (1994) Communication with parents of children with cancer. *Palliative Medicine* 8, 105–14.

Edgeworth, J., Bullock, P., Bailey, A., Gallagher, A. and Crouchman, M. (1996) Why are brain tumours still being missed? *Archives of Disease in Childhood* 74, 148–51.

Edwards, J., Gibson, F., Richardson, A. and Sepion, B.R.E. (2003) Fatigue in adolescents with and following a cancer diagnosis: developing and evidence base for practice. *European Journal of Cancer* 39, 2671–80.

Eiser, C., Greco, V. and Vance, Y. (2004) Perceived discrepancies and their resolution: quality of life in survivors of childhood cancer. *Psychology and Health* 19, 15–28.

Eiser, C., Havermans, T., Eiser, J. R. (1995) Parents' attributions about childhood cancer: implications for relationships with medical staff. *Child Care Health and Development* 21, 31–42.

Eiser, C., Hill, J. and Blacklay, A. (2000a) Surviving cancer; what does it mean for you? An evaluation of a clinic based intervention for survivors of childhood cancer. *Psycho-Oncology* 9, 214–20.

Eiser, C., Hill, J. and Vance, Y. (2000b) Examining the psychological consequences of surviving childhood cancer: systematic review as a research method in pediatric psychology. *Journal of Pediatric Psychology* 25, 449–60.

Eiser, C. and Morse, R. (2001a) Quality of life measures in chronic diseases of childhood. *Health Technology Assessment* 5, 1–157.

Eiser, C. and Morse, R. (2001b) A review of measures of quality of life for children with chronic illness. *Archives of Disease in Childhood* 84, 205–11.

Eiser, C., Parkyn, T., Havermans, T. and McNinch, A. (1994) Parents recall on the diagnosis of cancer in their child. *Psycho-Oncology* 3, 197–203.

Eiser, C., Vance, Y., Horne, B., Glaser, A. and Galvin, H. (2003) The value of PedsQLTM in assessing quality of life in survivors of childhood cancer. *Child: Care, Health and Development* 29, 95–102.

Ellis, R. and Leventhal, B. (1993) Information needs and decision-making preferences of children with cancer. *Psycho-Oncology* 2, 277–84.

Enskar, K., Carlsson, M., Golsater, M. and Hamrin, E. (1997a) Symptom distress and life situation in adolescents with cancer. *Cancer Nursing* 20, 23–33.

Enskar, K., Carlsson, M., Golsater, M., Hamrin, E. and Kreuger, A. (1997b) Life situation and problems as reported by children with cancer and their parents. *Journal of Pediatric Oncology Nursing* 14, 18–26.

Enskar, K., Carlsson, M., von Essen, L., Kreuger, A. and Hamrin, E. (1997c) Development of a tool to measure the life situation of parents of children with cancer. Quality of Life Research 6, 248–56.

Entwistle, V. (2000) Supporting and resourcing treatment decision-making: some policy considerations. *Health Expectations* 3, 77–85.

Erikson, J. (2004) Fatigue in adolescents with cancer: a review of the literature. *Clinical Journal of Oncology Nursing* 8, 139–45.

Evans, S. and Radford, M. (1995) Current lifestyle of young adults treated for cancer in childhood. *Archives of Disease in Childhood* 72, 423–6.

Faulkner, A., Peace, G. and O'Keeffe, C. (1995) *When a Child has Cancer.* London: Chapman & Hall.

Felder-Puig, R., Formann, A., Mildener, A., Feltblower, R., Lewis, I., Picton, S., Richards, M., Glaser, A., Kinsey, S. and McKinney, P. (1998) Quality of life and psychosocial adjustment of young patients after treatment of bone cancer. *Cancer* 83, 69–75.

Feltbower, R., Lewis, I., Picton, S., Richards, M., Glaser, A., Kinsey, S. and McKinney, P. (2004) Diagnosing childhood cancer in primary care – a realistic expectation? *British Journal of Cancer* 90, 1882–4.

Festa, R., Tamaroff, M., Chasalow, F. and Lanzkowsky, P. (1992) Therapeutic adherence to oral medication regimens by adolescents with cancer. I. Laboratory assessment. *The Journal of Pediatrics* 120, 807–11.

Fife, B., Norton, J. and Groom, G. (1987) The family's adaptation to childhood leukaemia. *Social Science and Medicine* 24, 159–68.

Fine, G. A. (2004) Adolescence as cultural toolkit: high school debate and the repertoires of childhood and adulthood. *Sociological Quarterly* 45, 1–20.

Frank, A. (1995) *The Wounded Story Teller: Body, Illness and Ethics.* Chicago: Chicago University Press.

Frank, N., Brown, R., Blount, R., Bunke, V. (2001) Predictors of affective responses of mothers and fathers of children with cancer. *Psycho-Oncology* 10, 293–304.

Frankenberg, R., Robinson, I. and Delahooke, A. (2000) Countering essentialism in behavioural social science: the example of 'the vulnerable child' examined. *The Sociological Review* 48, 586–611.

Fraser, D. (2003) Strangers in their own land: friendship issues when children have cancer. *Journal of Research in Special Educational Needs* 3, 147–53.

Freeman, K., O'Dell, C. and Meola, C. (2000) Issues in families of children with brain tumours. *Oncology Nursing Forum* 27, 843–8.

Freeman, M. (1997) *The Moral Status of Children: Essays on the Rights of the Child.* Dordrecht, The Netherlands: Kluwer.

Freeman, M. (1998) The sociology of childhood and children's rights. *The International Journal of Children's Rights* 6, 433–44.

Friedman, D. and Meadows, A. (2002) Late effects of childhood cancer therapy. *Pediatric Clinics of North America* 49, 1083–106.

Gabe, J., Olumide, G. and Bury, M. (2004) 'It takes three to tango': a framework for understanding patient partnership in paediatric clinics. *Social Science and Medicine* 59, 1071–9.

Gagnon, E. and Recklitis, C. (2003) Parents' decision-making preferences in pediatric-oncology: the relationship to health care involvement and complementary therapy use. *Psycho-Oncology* 12, 442–52.

Gatta, G., Capocaccia, R., De Angelis, R., Stiller, C. and Coebergh, J. (2003) Cancer survival in European adolescents and young adults. *European Journal of Cancer* 39, 2600–10.

Giddens, A. (1979) *Central Problems in Social Theory*. London: Macmillan.

Giddens, A. (1984) *The Constitution of Society: Outline of the Theory of Structuration*. Cambridge: Polity Press.

Giddens, A. (1991) *Modernity and Self-identity*. Cambridge: Polity Press.

Goffman, E. (1959) *The Presentation of the Self in Everyday Life*. New York: Doubleday Anchor.

Goffman, E. (1967) *Interaction Ritual: Essays on Face-to-face Behaviour*. New York: Doubleday Anchor.

Goffman, E. (1968) *Stigma: Notes on the Management of Spoiled Identity*. Harmondsworth: Penguin.

Goldenberg Libov, B., Nevid, J., Pelcovitz, D. and Carmony, T. (2002) Posttraumatic stress symtomatology in mothers of pediatric cancer survivors. *Psychology and Health* 17, 501–11.

Goodenough, T., Williamson, E., Kent, E. and Ashcroft, R. (2003) What did you think about that? Researching children's perceptions of participation in a longitudinal genetic epidemiology study. *Children and Society* 17, 113–25.

Gordon, G., Wallace, S. and Neal, J. (1995) Intracranial tumours during the first two years of life: presenting features. *Archives of Disease in Childhood* 73, 345–7.

Goswami, U. (2002a) *Blackwell Handbook of Childhood Cognitive Development*. Oxford: Blackwell Publishing.

Goswami, U. (2002b) Models of cognitive development, in Goswami, U., *Blackwell Handbook of Childhood Cognitive Development*. Oxford: Blackwell Publishing.

Gray, R., Doan, B., Shermer, P., FitzGerald, A., Berry, M., Jenkin, D. and Dohenty, M. (1992) Psychologic adaptation of survivors of childhood cancer. *Cancer* 70, 2713–21.

Green, D., Hyland, A., Bracos, M., Reynolds, J., Lee, R., Hall, B. and Zevon, M. (2000) Second malignant neoplasms after treatment for Hodgkin's disease in childhood or adolescence. *Journal of Clinical Oncology* 18, 1492–9.

Green, D., Zevon, M. and Hall, R. (1991) Achievement of life goals by adult survivors of modern treatment for childhood cancer. *Cancer* 67, 206–13.

Greig, A. and Taylor, J. (1999) *Doing Research with Children*. London: Sage.

Grinyer, A. and Thomas, C. (2001) Young adults with cancer: the effect of the illness on parents and families. *International Journal of Palliative Nursing* 7, 162–70.

Grootenhuis, M. and Last, B. (1997) Adjustment and coping by parents of children with cancer: a review of the literature. *Supportive Care in Cancer* 5, 466–84.

Grootenhuis, M. and Last, B. (2001) Children with cancer with different survival perspectives: defensiveness, control strategies and psychological adjustment. *Psycho-Oncology* 10, 305–14.

Gwyn, R. (2002) *Communicating Health and Illness*. London: Sage.

Gwyn, R., Elwyn, G., Edwards, A. and Mooney, A. (2003) The problematic of decision-sharing: deconstructing 'cholesterol' in a clinical encounter. *Health Expectations* 6, 242–54.

Haase, J. E. and Phillips, C. R. (2004) The adolescent/young adult experience. *Journal of Pediatric Oncology Nursing* 21, 145–9.

Haase, J. and Rostad, M. (1994) Experiences of completing cancer therapy: children perspectives. *Oncology Nursing Forum* 21, 1483–94.

Hagger, L. (2004) The Human Rights Act 1998 and medical treatment: time for re-examination. *Archives of Disease in Childhood* 89, 460–3.

Haimi, M., Peretz Nahum, M. and Weyl Ben Arush, M. (2004) Delay in diagnosis of children with cancer: a retrospective study of 315 children. *Pediatric Hematology and Oncology* 21, 37–48.

Halperin, E., Watson, D. and George, S. (2001) Duration of symptoms prior to diagnosis is related inversely to presenting disease stage in children with medulloblastoma. *Cancer* 91, 1444–50.

Hamre, M., Williams, J., Chuba, P., Bhambhani, K., Ravindranath, Y. and Severson, R. (2000) Early deaths in childhood cancer. *Medical and Pediatric Oncology* 34, 343–7.

Harden, J., Scott, S., Backett-Milburn, K. and Jackson, S. (2000) Can't talk, won't talk? Methodological issues in researching children. *Sociological Research Online* 5.

Harder, L. and Bowditch, C. (1982) Siblings of children with cystic fibrosis: perceptions of the impact of the disease. *Children's Health Care* 10, 116–20.

Harris, P. (1989) *Children and Emotion*. Hove: Erlbaum.

Haupt, R., Fears, T., Robinson, L., Mills, J., Nichdson, H., Zeltzer, L., Meadows, A. and Byrne, J. (1994) Educational attainment in long-term survivors of acute lymphoblastic leukaemia. *Journal of the American Medical Association* 272, 1427–32.

Hays, D. (1993) Adult survivors of childhood cancer. employment and insurance issues in different age groups. *Cancer* 71, 3306–9.

Hedstrom, M., Haglund, K., Skolin, I. and Von Essen, L. (2003) Distressing events for children and adolescents with cancer: child, parent and nurse perceptions. *Journal of Pediatric Oncology Nursing* 20, 120–32.

Hergenrather, J. and Rabinowitz, M. (1991) Age-related differences in the organisation of children's knowledge of illness. *Developmental Psychology* 27, 952–9.

Hicks, J., Bartholomew, J. and Ward-Smith, P. (2003) Quality of life among childhood leukaemia patients. *Journal of Pediatric Oncology Nursing* 20, 192–200.

Hill, J., Kondryn, H., Mackie, E., McNally, R. and Eden, T. (2003) Adult psychosocial functioning following childhood cancer: the different roles of sons' and daughters' relationships with their fathers and mothers. *Journal of Child Psychology and Psychiatry* 44, 752–62.

Hinds, P., Hockenberry-Eaton, M., Gilger, E., Kline, N., Burleson, C., Bottomley, S. and others (1999) Comparing patient, parent and staff descriptions of fatigue in pediatric oncology patients. *Cancer Nursing* 22, 277–89.

Hinds, P. and Martin, J. (1988) Hopefulness and the self-sustaining process in adolescents with cancer. *Nursing Research* 37, 336–40.

Hockenberry-Eaton, M. (1994) Living with cancer: children with extraordinary courage. *Oncology Nursing Forum* 21, 1025–31.

Hockenberry-Eaton, M., Hinds, P., Alcoser, P., O'Neill, J., Enell, K., Howard, V., Gattuso, J. and Taylor, J. (1998) Fatigue in children and adolescents with cancer. *Journal of Pediatric Oncology Nursing* 15, 172–82.

Hockenberry-Eaton, M. and Minick, P. (1994) Living with cancer: Children with extraordinary courage. *Oncology Nursing Forum* 21, 1025–31.

Holm, K., Patterson, J. and Gurney, J. (2003) Parental involvement and family-centred care in the diagnostic and treatment phases of childhood cancer: results from a qualitative study. *Journal of Pediatric Oncology Nursing* 20, 301–13.

Holstein, J. and Miller, G. (1990) Rethinking victimization: an interactional approach to victimology. *Symbolic Interaction* 13, 103–22.

Holt, J. (1975) *Escape from Childhood*. Hardmondsworth: Penguin.

Horowitz, W. and Kazak, A. (1990) Family adaptation to childhood cancer: sibling and family system variables. *Journal of Clinical Child Psychology* 19, 221–8.

Houtzager, B., Grootenhuis, M., Hoekstra-Weebers, J., Caron, H. and Last, B. (2003) Psychosocial functioning in siblings with paediatric cancer patients one to six months after diagnosis. *European Journal of Cancer* 39, 1423–32.

Houtzager, B., Grootenhuis, M. and Last, B. (1999) Adjustment of siblings to childhood cancer: a literature review. *Supportive Care in Cancer* 7, 302–20.

Hudson, M., Mertens, A., Yasui, Y., Hobbie, W., Chen, H., Gurney, J., Yeazel, M., Recklitis, C., Marina, N., Robison, L. and Oeffinger, K. (2003) Health status of adult long-term survivors of childhood cancer: a report from the Childhood Cancer Survivor Study. *JAMA* 290, 1583–92.

Hutchby, I. and Moran-Ellis, J. (1998a) Children and social competence: arenas of action. London: Falmer.

Hutchby, I. and Moran-Ellis, J. (1998b) Situating children's social competence. Hutchby, I and Moran-Ellis, J. Children and social competence: arenas of action. London: Falmer.

Hyden, L. (1997) Illness and narrative. *Sociology of Health and Illness* 19, 48–69.

Ibrahim, K. A. R. (2004) Seizures as the presenting symptom if brain tumours in children. *Seizure* 13, 108–112.

Inman, C. (1991) Analysed interaction in a children's oncology clinic: the child's view and the parent's opinion of the effect of medical encounters. *Journal of Advanced Nursing* 16, 782–93.

Institute of Medicine (2003) *Childhood Cancer Survivorship: Improving Care and Quality of Life.* Washington: National Academy of Sciences.

James, A. and James, A. (2001a) Childhood: toward a theory of continuity and change. *Annals of the American Academy of Political and Social Science* 575, 25–37.

James, A. and James A. (2001b) Tightening the net: children, community and control. *British Journal of Sociology* 52, 211–28.

James, A. and James, A. (2004) *Constructing Childhood.* Basingstoke: Palgrave Macmillan.

James, A., Jenks, C. and Prout, A. (1998) *Theorizing Childhood.* Cambridge: Polity Press.

James, K., Keegan-Wells, D., Hinds, P., Kelly, K., Bond, D., Hall, B., Mahan, R., Moore, I., Roll, L. and Speckhart, B. (2002) The care of my child with cancer: parents perceptions of caregiving demands. *Journal of Pediatric Oncology Nursing* 19, 218–28.

James, A. and Prout, A. (1990) *Constructing and Reconstructing Childhood: Contemporary Issues in the Sociological Study of Childhood.* London: Falmer Press.

James, A. and Prout, A. (1996) Strategies and structures: towards a new perspective on children's experiences of family life, in O'Brien, J. and O'Brien, M., *Children in Families: Research and Policy.* London: Falmer.

Jenks, C. (1996a) *Childhood.* London: Routledge.

Jenks, C. (1996b) The postmodern child, in Brannen, J. and O'Brien, M., *Children in Families: Research and Policy.* London: Falmer Press.

Jones, J. and Neil-Urban, S. (2003) Father to father: focus groups of fathers of children with cancer. *Social Work in Health Care* 37, 41–61.

Kadan-Lottick, N., Robison, L., Gurney, J., Neglia, JP, Yasui, Y., Hayashi, R., Hudson, M., Greenberg, M. and Mertens, A. (2002) Childhood cancer survivors' knowledge about their past diagnosis and treatment: Childhood Cancer Survivor Study. *JAMA* 287, 1832–9, 1875–6.

Kagan, J. (2003) Biology, context and developmental inquiry. *Annual Review of Psychology* 54, 1–23.

Kalapurakal, J., Dome, J., Perlman, E., Malogolowkin, M., Haase, G., Grundy, P. and Coppes, M. (2004) Management of Wilms' tumour: current practice and future goals. *Lancet Oncology* 5, 37–46.

Kalish, C. (1996) Causes and symptoms in preschoolers' conceptions of illness. *Child Development* 67, 1647–70.

Kameny, R. and Bearison, D. (2002) Cancer narratives of adolescents and young adults: a qualitative and quantitative analysis. *Children's Health Care* 3, 143–73.

Karian, V., Jankowski, S. and Beal, J. (1998) Exploring the lived-experience of childhood cancer survivors. *Journal of Pediatric Oncology Nursing* 15, 153–62.

Kazak, A., Stuber, M., Barakat, L., Meeske, K., Guthrie, D. and Meadows, A. (1998) Predicting posttraumatic stress symptoms in mothers and fathers of survivors of childhood cancers. *Journal of the American Academy of Child and Adolescent Psychiatry* 37, 823–31.

Kazak, A. and Barakat, L. (1997) Brief report: parenting stress and quality of life during treatment for childhood leukaemia predicts child and parent adjustment after treatment ends. *Journal of Pediatric Psychology* 22, 749–58.

Kazak, A., Barakat, L., Meeske, K., Christakis, D., Meadows, A., Casey, R., Penati, B. and Stuber, M. (1997) Posttraumatic stress, family functioning, and social support in survivors of childhood leukaemia and their mothers and fathers. *Journal of Consulting and Clinical Psychology* 65, 120–9.

Kazak, A., Cant, C., Jensen, M., McSherry, M., Rourke, M., Hwang, W., Alderfer, M., Beele, D., Simms, S and Lange, B. (2003) Identifying psychosocial risk indicative of subsequent resource use in families of newly diagnosed pediatric oncology patients. *Journal of Clinical Oncology* 21, 3220–5.

Kelly, D., Pearce, S. and Mulhall, A. (2004) 'Being in the same boat': ethnographic insights into an adolescent cancer unit. *International Journal of Nursing Studies*, 847–57.

Kelly, M. (1986) The subjective experience of chronic disease: some implications of the management of ulcerative colitis. *Journal of Chronic Disease* 39, 653–66.

Kennard, B., Stewart, S., Olvera, R., Bawdon, R. and OhAilin, A. (2004) Non adherence in adolescent oncology patients: preliminary data on psychological risk factors and relationships to outcome. *Journal of Clinical Psychology in Medical Settings* 11, 31–9.

Kennedy, I. and Grubb, A. (2000) *Medical Law*. London: Butterworths.

Koch-Hattem, A. (1986) Siblings's experience of pediatric cancer: interviews with children. *Health and Social Work* 11, 107–11.

Koch, T. (2000) The illusion of paradox. *Social Science and Medicine* 50, 757–9.

Koocher, G. and O'Malley, J. (1981) *The Damocles Syndrome: Psychosocial Consequences of Childhood Cancer*. New York: McGraw-Hill.

Kramer, R. (1984) Living with childhood cancer: impact on healthy siblings. *Oncology Nursing Forum* 11, 44–51.

Kupst, M., Natta, M., Richardson, C., Schulman, J., Lavigine, J. and Das, L. (1995) Family coping with pediatric leukaemia: ten years after treatment. *Journal of Pediatric Psychology* 20, 601–17.

Kvist, S., Rajanthe, J., Kvist, M., and Siimes, M. (1991) Perceptions of problematic events and quality of care among patients after successful therapy of the child's malignant disease. *Social Science and Medicine* 33, 249–56.

Lancaster, D., Lennard, L. and Lilleyman, J. (1997) Profile of non-compliance in lymphoblastic leukaemia. *Archives of Disease in Childhood* 76, 365–6.

Landolt, M., Vollrath, M. and Ribi, K. (2002) Predictors of coping strategy selection in paediatric patients. *Acta Paediatrica* 91, 954–60.

Landolt, M., Vollrath, M., Ribi, K., Gnehm, H. and Sennhauser, F. (2003) Incidence and associations of parental and child posttraumatic stress symptoms in pediatric patients. *Journal of Child Psychology and Psychiatry* 44, 1199–207.

Langeveld, N., Grootenhuis, M., Voute, P., De Haan, R. and van den Bos, C. (2004) Quality of life, self-esteem and worries in young adult survivors of childhood cancer. *Psycho-Oncology*, 13: 867–81.

Langeveld, N., Ubbink, M. C. and Last, B. (2003) Educational achievement, employment and living situation in long-term survivors of childhood cancer in the Netherlands. *Psycho-Oncology* 12, 213–25.

Lansdown, G. Children's rights. Mayall, B. (1994) *Children's Childhoods Observed and Experienced*. London: Falmer.

Lansky, S., List, M., Ritter-Sterr, C. (1986) Psychosocial consequences of cure. *Cancer* 58, 529–33.

Last, B. and van Veldhuizen, A. (1996) Information about diagnosis and prognosis related to anxiety and depression in children with cancer aged 8–16 years. *European Journal of Cancer* 32A, 290–4.

Lee, N. (2001) *Childhood and Society, Growing up in an Age of Uncertainty*. Buckingham: Open University Press.

Lesko, N. (1996) Denaturalizing adolescence: the politics of contemporary representations. *Youth and Society* 28, 139–61.

Lesko, N. (2001) *Act your Age: A Cultural Construction of Adolescence*. New York: Routledge Inc.

Levenson, P., Pfefferbaum, B., Copeland, D. and Silberg, Y. (1982) Information preferences of cancer patients ages 11–20. *Journal of Adolescent Health* 3, 9–13.

Levi, R., Marsick, R., Drotar, D. and Kodish, E. (2000) Diagnosis, disclosure, and informed consent: learning from parents of children with cancer. *Journal of Pediatric Hematology and Oncology* 22, 3–12.

Leydon, G., Boulton, M., Moynihan, C., Jones, A., Mossman, J., Boudioni, M. and McPherson, K. (2000) Cancer patients' information needs and information seeking behaviour: in depth interview study. *British Medical Journal* 320, 909–13.

Little, M., Paul, K., Jordens, C. and Sayers, E. (2002) Survivorship and discourses of identity. *Psycho-Oncology* 11, 170–8.

Little, M., Paul, K., Jordens, C. F. C. and Sayers, E. J. (2000) Vulnerability in the narratives of patients and their carers: studies of colorectal cancer. *Health* 4, 495–510.

Little, M. and Sayers, E. (2004) While there's life . . . hope and experience of cancer. *Social Science and Medicine* 59, 1329–37.

Ljungman, G., Gordh, T., Sorensen, S. and Kreuger, A. (1999) Pain in paediatric oncology: interviews with children, adolescents and their parents. *Acta Paediatrica* 88, 623–30.

Lowden, J. (2002) Children's rights: a decade of dispute. *Journal of Advanced Nursing* 37, 100–7.

Lozowski, S. (1993) Views of childhood cancer survivors. *Cancer* 71, 3354–7.

Lähteenmäki, P., Huostila, J. and Hinkka, S. (2002) Childhood cancer patients at school. *European Journal of Cancer* 38, 1227–40.

Lupton, D. and Barclay, L. (1997) *Constructing Fatherhood: Discourses and Experiences*. London: Sage.

Mackie, E., Hill, J., Kondryn, H. and McNally, R. (2000) Adult psychosocial outcomes in long-term survivors of acute lymphoblastic leukaemia and Wilms' tumour: a controlled study. *Lancet* 355, 1310–14.

Mackie, E., Radford, M. and Shalet, S. (1996) Gonadal function following chemotherapy for childhood Hodgkin's disease. *Medical and Pediatric Oncology* 27, 74–8.

Madan-Swain, A., Brown, R., Sexson, S., Baldwin, K., Pais, R. and Ragab, A. (1994) Adolescent cancer survivors: psychosocial and familial adaptation. *Psychosomatics* 35, 453–9.

Manne, S., Lesanics, D., Meyers, P., Wollner, N., Steinherz, P. and Redd, W. (1995) Predictors of depressive symtomatology among parents of newly diagnosed children with cancer. *Journal of Pediatric Psychology* 20, 491–510.

Manning, P. (1992) *Erving Goffman and Modern Sociology. Cambridge*: Polity Press.

Martinson, I. and Cohen, M. (1988) Themes from a longitudinal study of family reaction to childhood cancer. *Journal of Psychosocial Oncology* 6, 81–98.

Martinson, I., Gillis, C., Colaizzo, D., Freeman, M. and Bassert, E. (1990) Impact of childhood cancer on healthy school age siblings. *Cancer Nursing* 13, 183–90.

Massimo, L. (2004) From informed consent to shared consent: a developing process in paediatric oncology. *Lancet Oncology* 5, 384–7.

Mathieson, C. and Stam, H. (1995) Renegotiating identity: cancer narratives. *Sociology of Health and Illness* 17, 283–306.

Mauthner, M. (1997) Methodological aspects of collecting data from children: lessons from three research projects. *Children and Society* 11, 16–28.

Mayall, B. (1994a) *Children's Childhoods: Observed and Experienced*. London: Falmer Press.

Mayall, B. (1994b) Introduction, in Mayall, B., *Children's Childhoods Observed and Experienced*. London: Falmer.

Mayall, B. (1996) *Children, Health and the Social Order*. Buckingham: Open University Press.

Mayall, B. (1998) Towards a sociology of child health. *Sociology of Health and Illness* 20, 269–88.

Mayall, B. (2000) The sociology of childhood in relation to children's rights. *The International Journal of Children's Rights* 8, 243–59.

Mayall, B. (2002) *Towards a Sociology for Childhood: Thinking from Children's Lives.* Buckingham: Open University Press.

McGarrigle, J. and Donaldson, M. (1974) Conservation accidents. *Cognition* 3, 341–50.

McGrath, P. and Pitcher, L. (2002) 'Enough is enough': qualitative findings on the impact of dexamethasone during reinduction/consolidation for paediatric acute lymphoblastic leukaemia. *Supportive Cancer Care* 10, 146–55.

McHale, J., Fox, M. and Murphy, J. (1997) *Health Care Law.* London: Sweet & Maxwell.

McHale, J. and Gallagher, A. (2003) *Nursing and Human Rights.* Edinburgh: Butterworth Heinemann.

McHale, J. and Tingle, J. (2001) *Law and Nursing.* Oxford: Butterworth Heinemann.

McKeever, P. and Miller, K. (2004) Mothering children who have disabilities: a Bourdieusian interpretation of maternal practices. *Social Science and Medicine* 59, 1177–91.

Meloff, K. (1982) Headaches in children. Cause for parental concern but commonly benign. *Postgraduate Medicine* 72, 195–9, 202.

Miles, R. (2000) The GP strategy for headaches in children. *Practitioner* 244, 618–22, 625–6.

Mitby, P., Robinson, L., Whitton, J., Zevon, M., Gibbs, I., Tersak, J., Meadows, A., Stovall, M., Zeltzer, L. and Mertens, A., Childhood Cancer Survivor Study Steering Committee (2003) Utilization of special education services and educational attainment among long-term survivors of childhood cancer. *Cancer* 97, 115–26.

Moller, D. (1996) *Confronting Death: Values, Institutions and Human Mortality.* Oxford: Oxford University Press.

Morss, J. (2002) The several constructions of James, Jenks and Prout: a contribution to the sociological theorisation of childhood. *International Journal of Children's Rights* 10, 39–54.

Moss, P., Dillon, J. and Statham, J. (2000) The 'child in need' and 'the rich child': discourses, constructions and practice. *Critical Social Policy* 20, 233–54.

Mulhern, R., Merchant, T., Gajjar, A., Reddick, W. and Kun, L. (2004) Late neurocognitive sequelae in survivors of brain tumours in childhood. *Lancet Oncology* 5, 399–408.

Murray, J. (2002) A qualitative exploration of psychosocial support for siblings of children with cancer. *Journal of Pediatric Nursing* 17, 327–37.

Neff, K. and Helwig, C. (2002) A constructivist approach to understanding the development of reasoning about rights and authority within cultural contexts. *Cognitive Development* 17, 1429–50.

Noll, R., Bukowski, W., Davies, W., Koontz, K. and Kulkani, R. (1993) Adjustment in the peer system of adolescents with cancer: a two year study. *Journal of Pediatric Psychology* 18, 351–64.

Noll, R., Garstein, M., Vannatta, K., Corell, J., Bukowski, W. and Davies, W. (1999)

Social, emotional and behavioural functioning of children with cancer. *Pediatrics* 103, 71–8.

Norberg, A., Lindblad, F. and Boman, K. (2005) Coping strategies in parents of children with cancer. *Social Science and Medicine* 60, 965–75.

Nygaard, R., Clausen, N., Siimes, M., Marky, I., Skjeldestad, F., Kristinsson, J., Vuoristo, A., Wegelius, R. and Moe, P. (1991) Reproduction following treatment for childhood leukaemia: a population-based prospective cohort study of fertility and offspring. *Medical and Pediatric Oncology* 19, 459–66.

O'Kane, C. (2000) The development of participatory techniques: facilitating children's views about decisions which affect them, in Christensen, P. and James, A., *Research with Children: Perspectives and Practices*. London: RoutledgeFalmer.

Oakley, A. (1994) Women and children first and last: parallels and differences between children's and women's studies, in Mayall, B., *Children's Childhoods Observed and Experienced*. London: Falmer.

Ornstein, P., Baker-Ward, L., Gordon, B. and Meritt, K. (1997) Children's memory for medical experiences: implications for testimony. *Applied Cognitive Psychology* 11, 107.

Parkin, D., Kramarova, E., Draper, G., Masuyer, E., Michelis, J., Neglia, J., Quereshi, S. and Stiller, C. (1998) *International Incidence of Childhood Cancer*, Vol II. 144. International Agency for Research on Cancer: Lyons, IACR Scientific Publications.

Parry, C. (2003) Embracing uncertainty: an exploration of the experiences of childhood cancer survivors. *Qualitative Health Research* 13, 227–46.

Patistea, E., Makrodimitri, P. and Panteli, V. (2000) Greek parents' reactions, difficulties and resources in childhood leukaemia at the time of diagnosis. *European Journal of Cancer Care* 9, 86–96.

Patterson, J., Holm, K. and Gurney, J. (2004) The impact of childhood cancer on the family: a qualitative analysis of statins, resources, and coping behaviours. *Psycho-Oncology* 13, 390–407.

Pendley, J., Dahlquist, L. and Dreyer, Z. (1997) Body image and psychosocial adjustment in adolescent cancer survivors. *Journal of Pediatric Psychology* 22, 29–43.

Perrin, E. and Gerrity, S. (1981) There's a demon in your belly: children's understandings of illness. *Pediatrics* 67, 841–9.

Perrin, E., Lewkowicz, C. and Young, M. (2000) Shared vision: concordance among fathers, mothers, and pediatricians about the unmet needs of children with chronic health conditions. *Pediatrics* 105 277–85.

Peterson, C. and Rideout, R. (1998) Memory for medical emergencies experienced by 1- and 2-year olds. *Developmental Psychology* 34, 1059–72.

Peterson, C. and Siegal, M. (1999) Competence to consent, in Siegal, M. and Peterson, C. C., *Children's Understanding of Biology and Health*, 257–79. Cambridge: Cambridge University Press.

Phipps, S. (1999) Approaches to the measurement of depressive symptomatology in children with cancer: attempting to circumvent the effects of defensiveness. *Journal of Developmental and Behavioural Pediatrics* 20, 150–6.

Pill, R. and Stott, N. (1982) Concepts of illness causation and responsibility: some preliminary data from a sample of working class mothers. *Social Science and Medicine* 16, 43–52.

Pinkerton, C. and Plowman, P. (1997) *Clinical Practice and Controversies*. London: Chapman & Hall Medical.

Pole, C., Mizen, P. and Bolton, A. (1999) Realising children's agency in research: partners and participants? *International Journal of Social Research Methodology* 2, 39–54.

Pollock, B., Krischer, J. and Vietti, T. (1991) Interval between symptom onset and diagnosis of pediatric solid tumors. *Journal of Pediatrics* 119, 725–32.

Prout, A. (2000) *The Body, Childhood and Society*. Basingstoke: Macmillan.

Prout, A. and James, A. (1997) A new paradigm for the sociology of childhood? Provenance, promise and problems, in James, A. and Prout, A. (eds) *Constructing and Reconstructing Childhood*. London: Falmer.

Pui, C., Cheng, C., Leung, W., Rai, S., Rivera, G., Sandlund, J., Ribeiro, R., Relling, M., Kun, L., Evans, W. and Hudson, M. (2003) Extended follow-up of long-term survivors of childhood acute lymphoblastic leukaemia. *New England Journal of Medicine* 349, 640–9.

Pyke-Grimm, K., Degner, L., Small, A. and Mueller, B. (1999) Preferences for participation in treatment decision making and information needs of parents with cancer: a pilot study. *Journal of Pediatric Oncology* 16, 13–24.

Qvortrup, J. (1994) Childhood matters: an introduction, in Qvortrup, J., Bardy, M., Sgritta, G. and Wintersberger, H., *Childhood Matters: Social Theory Practice and Politics*. Aldershot: Avebury.

Qvortrup, J. (1997) A voice for children in statistical and social accounting: a plea for children's right to be heard, in James, A. and Prout, A., *Constructing and Reconstructing Childhood*. London: Falmer.

Qvortrup, J., Bardy, M., Sgritta, G. and Wintersberger, H. (1994) *Childhood Matters: Social Theory, Practice and Politics*. Aldershot: Avebury.

Reay, D., Bignold, S., Ball, S. and Cribb, A. (1998) 'He just had a different way of showing it': gender dynamics in families coping with childhood cancer. *Journal of Gender Studies* 7, 39–52.

Rechner, M. (1990) Adolescents with cancer: getting on with life. *Journal of Pediatric Oncology Nursing* 7, 139–44.

Reiter-Purtill, J., Vannatta, K., Gerhardt, C. and others (2003) A controlled study of the social functioning of children who completed treatment of cancer. *Journal of Pediatric Hematology and Oncology* 25, 467–73.

Ressler, I., Cash, J., McNeill, D., Joy, S. and Rosoff, P. (2003) Continued parental attendance at a clinic for adult survivors of childhood cancer. *Journal of Pediatric Hematology and Oncology* 25, 868–73.

Richardson, D. (1993) *Women, Mothering and Childrearing.* Basingstoke: Macmillan.

Roche, J. (1996) The politics of children's rights, in Brannen, J. and O'Brien, M., *Children in Families: Research and Policy.* London: Falmer Press.

Roche, J. (1999) Children: rights, participation and citizenship. *Childhood* 6, 475–93.

Rolland, J. (1997) The meaning of disability and suffering: sociopolitical and ethical concerns. *Family Process* 36, 437–40.

Ross, L., Johansen, C., Dalton, S., Meltemkjaer, L., Thomassen, L., Mortensen, P. and Olsen, J. (2003) Psychiatric hospitalizations among survivors of cancer in childhood or adolescence. *New England Journal of Medicine* 349, 650–57.

Ross, L. (1997) Health care decision making by children – is it in their best interest? *The Hastings Center Report* 27, 41–5.

Rowe, S. and Wertsch, J. (2002) Vygotsky's model of cognitive development, in Goswami, U., *Blackwell Handbook of Childhood Cognitive Development,* 538–54. Oxford: Blackwell Publishing.

Royal College of Paediatrics and Child Health (2000) *Advocating for Children.* London: RCPCH.

Rushforth, H. (1999) Practitioner review: communicating with hospitalised children: review and application of research pertaining to children's understanding of health and illness. *Journal of Child Psychology and Psychiatry* 40, 683–91.

Rutter, M. (2000) Psychosocial influences: critiques, findings, and research needs. *Developmental Psychopathology* 12, 375–405.

Saha, V., Love, S., Eden, T., Micallef-Eynaud, P. and MacKinlay, G. (1993) Determinants of symptom interval in childhood cancer. *Archives of Disease in Childhood* 68, 771–4.

Saile, H., Burgmeier, R. and Schmidt, L. (1988) A meta-analysis of studies on psychological preparation of children facing medical procedures. *Psychology and Health* 2, 107–132.

Salmon, P. and Hall, G. (2003) Patient empowerment and control: a psychological discourse in the service of medicine. *Social Science and Medicine* 57, 1969–80.

Sawyer, M., Antoniou, G., Toogood, I. and Rice, M. (1997) Childhood cancer: a two-year prospective study of the psychological adjustment of children and parents. *Journal of the American Academy of Child and Adolescent Psychiatry* 36, 1736–49.

Sawyer, M., Antoniou, G., Toogood, I., Rice, M. and Baghurst, P. (2000) Childhood cancer: a 4-year prospective study of the psychological adjustment of children and parents. *Journal of Pediatric Hematology and Oncology* 22, 214–20.

Sawyer, M., Streiner, D., Antoniou, G., Toogood, I. and Rice, M. (1998) Influence of parental and family adjustment on the later psychological adjustment of children treated for cancer. *Journal of the American Academy of Child and Adolescent Psychiatry* 37, 815–22.

Scambler, G. and Hopkins, A. (1986) Being epileptic: coming to terms with stigma. *Sociology of Health and Illness* 8, 26–43.

Schmidt, S., Petersen, C. and Bullinger, M. (2003) Coping with chronic disease from the perspective of children and adolescents – a conceptual framework and its implications for participation. *Child: Care, Health and Development* 29, 63–75.

Schutz, A. (1962) *Collected Papers I: The Problem of Social Reality.* The Hague: Martinus Nijhoff.

Schutz, A. (1964) *Collected Papers II: Studies in Social Theory.* The Hague: Martinus Nijhoff.

Schutz, A. (1966) *Collected Papers III: Studies in Phenomenological Philosophy.* The Hague: Martinus Nijhoff.

Schwartz, C., Feinberg, R., Jilinskaia, E. and Applegate, J. (1999) An evaluation of a psychosocial intervention for survivors of childhood cancer: paradoxical effects of response shift over time. *Psycho-Oncology* 8, 344–54.

Sclater, D., Bainham, A. and Richards, M. (1999) Introduction, in Bainham, A., Sclater, D. A. and Richards, M., *What is a Parent? A Socio-legal Analysis.* Oxford: Hart.

Scott, J., Harmsen, M., Prictor, M., Sowden, A. and Watt, I. (2001) *Communicating with Children and Adolescents About their Cancer* [4]. Oxford: Update Software, Cochrane Library.

Scott, S., Jackson, S. and Backett-Milburn, K. (1998) Swings and roundabouts: risk anxiety and the everyday worlds of children. *Sociology* 32, 689–707.

Sharp, L. and Lipsky, M. (2002) Screening for depression across the lifespan: a review of measures for use in primary care settings. *American Family Physician* 66, 1001–8.

Sharpe, D. and Rossiter, L. (2002) Siblings of children with chronic illness: a meta-analysis. *Journal of Pediatric Psychology* 27, 699–710.

Shaw, I. (1996) Unbroken voices: children, young people and qualitative methods, in Butler, I. and Shaw, I., *A Case of Neglect? Children's Experiences and the Sociology of Childhood.* Aldershot: Avebury.

Siegal, M. and Peterson, C. (1996) Breaking the mold: a fresh look at children's understanding of questions about lies and mistakes. *Developmental Psychology* 32, 322–34.

Siegal, M. and Peterson, C. (1999) Becoming mindful of biology and health: an introduction, in Siegal, M. and Peterson, C. C., *Children's Understanding of Biology and Health*, Cambridge: Cambridge University Press.

Sillanpaa, M., Piekkala, P. and Kero, P. (1991) Prevalence of headache at preschool age in an unselected child population. *Cephalagia* 11, 239–42.

Silverman, D. (1987) Communication and medical practice: social relations and the clinic. London: Sage.

Silverman, D., Baker, C. and Keogh, J. (1998) The case of the silent child: advice giving and advice reception in parent-teacher interviews, in Hutchy, I.

and Moran-Ellis, J., *Children and Social Competence: Arenas of Action*. London: Falmer.

Simone, J. (2003) Childhood leukemia – successes and challenges for survivors. *New England Journal of Medicine* 349, 627–8.

Sloper, P. (1996) Needs and responses of parents following the diagnosis of childhood cancer. *Child: Care, Health and Development* 22, 187–202.

Sloper, P. (2000a) Experiences and support needs of siblings of children with cancer. *Health and Social Care in the Community* 8, 298–306.

Sloper, P. (2000b) Predictors of distress in parents of children with cancer: a prospective study. *Journal of Pediatric Psychology* 25, 79–91.

Sloper, P. and Turner, S. (1993) Risk and resistance factors in the adaptation of parents of children with severe physical disability. *Journal of Child Psychology and Psychiatry* 34, 167–88.

Sloper, P. and While, D. (1996) Risk factors in the adjustment of siblings of children with cancer. *Journal of Child Psychology and Psychiatry and Allied Disciplines* 37, 597–607.

Smith, L. (2002) Piaget's model, in Goswami, U., *Blackwell Handbook of Childhood Cognitive Development*, 515–37. Oxford: Blackwell Publishing.

Solberg, A. (1997) Negotiating childhood: changing constructions of age for Norwegian children, in James, A. and Prout, A., *Constructing and Reconstructing Childhood*. London: Falmer.

Spinetta, J. (1974) The dying child's awareness of death: a review. *Psychological Bulletin* 81, 259–60.

Spinetta, J. (1981) The sibling of the child with cancer, in Spinetta, J. J. and Deasy-Spinetta, P., *Living with Childhood Cancer*, 133–42. Mosby. St Louis.

Spinetta, J., Masera, G., Jankovic, M., Oppenheim, D., Martins, A., Ben Arush, M., van Dongen-Melman, J., Epelman, C., Medin, G., Pekkanen, K. and Eden, T. (2003) Valid informed consent and participative decision-making in children with cancer and their parents: a report of the SIOP Working Committee on psychosocial issues in pediatric oncology. *Medical and Pediatric Oncology* 40, 244–6.

Stacey, J. (1997) *Teratologies: A Cultural Study of Cancer*. London: Routledge.

Stainton Rogers, R. and Stainton Rogers, W. (1992) *Stories of Childhood: Shifting Agendas of Child Concern*. Hemel Hempstead: Harvester Wheatsheaf.

Stam, H., Grootenhuis, M. and Last, B. (2001) Social and emotional adjustment in young survivors of childhood cancer. *Supportive Cancer Care* 9, 489–513.

Sternberg, R. (2002) Individual differences in cognitive development, in Goswami, U., *Blackwell Handbook of Childhood Cognitive Development*, 600–19. Oxford: Blackwell Publishing.

Stevens, M., Mahler, H. and Parkes, S. (1998) The health status of adult survivors of cancer in childhood. *European Journal of Cancer* 34, 694–8.

Stewart, J. (2003) 'Getting used to it': children finding the ordinary and routine in the uncertainty context of cancer. *Qualitative Health Research* 13, 394–407.

Stiller, C., Quinn, M. and Rowan, S. (2004) *Childhood Cancer. The Health of Children and Young People*. London: Office of National Statistics.

Stiller, C. (2004) Epidemiology and genetics of childhood cancer. *Oncogene* 23, 6429–44.

Stiller, C., McKinney, P., Bunch, K., Bailey, C. and Lewis, I. (1991) Childhood cancer and ethnic group in Britain: a United Kingdom Children's Cancer Study Group (UKCCSG) study. *British Journal of Cancer* 64, 543–8.

Stokes, M. and Drake-Lee, A. (1998) Children who withdraw consent for elective surgery. *Paediatric Anaesthesia* 8, 113–15.

Storrie, T. (1997) Citizens or what, in Roche, J. and Tucker, S., *Youth and Society*. London: Sage/Open University.

Streisand, R., Braniecki, S., Tercyak, K. and Kazak, A. (2001) Childhood illness-related parenting stress: the pediatric inventory for parents. *Journal of Pediatric Psychology* 26, 155–62.

Strong, P. (1979) *The Ceremonial Order of the Clinic: Parents, Doctors and Medical Bureaucracies*. London: Routledge & Kegan Paul.

Strong, P. (1983) The importance of being Erving. Erving Goffman 1922–1982. *Sociology of Health and Illness* 5, 345–55.

Stuber, M., Christakis, D., Houskamp, B. and Kazak, A. (1996) Posttraumatic symptoms in childhood leukaemia survivors and their parents. *Psychosomatics* 37, 254–61.

Summerfield, D. (2001) The invention of post-traumatic stress disorder and the social usefulness of a psychiatric category. *British Medical Journal* 322, 95–8.

Swallow, V. and Jacoby, A. (2001) Mothers' evolving relationships with doctors and nurses during the chronic childhood illness trajectory, *Journal of Advanced Nursing* 36, 755–64.

Sweeting, H. and West, P. (1998) Health at age 11: reports from school children and their parents. *Archives of Disease in Childhood* 78, 427–34.

Taïeb, O., Moro, M., Baubet, T., Revah-Levy, A. and Flament, M. (2003) Post-traumatic stress symptoms after childhood cancer. *European Child and Adolescent Psychiatry* 12, 255–264.

Tait, A., Voepel-Lewis, T., Munro, H. and Malviya, S. (2001) Parents' preferences for participation in decisions made regarding their child's anaesthetic care. *Pediatric Anaesthesia* 11, 283–90.

Tates, K. and Meeuwesen, L. (2001) Doctor–parent–child communication. A (re)-view of the literature. *Social Science and Medicine* 52, 839–51.

Tates, K., Meeuwesen, L., Elbers, E. and Bensing, J. (2002) 'I've come for his throat': roles and identities in doctor–parent–child communication. *Child: Care, Health and Development* 28, 109–16.

Tates, K. M. L. and Meeuwersen, L. (2000) 'Let mum have her say': turntaking in doctor–parent–child communication. *Patient Education and Counseling* 40, 151–62.

Thulesius, H., Pola, J. and Hakansson, A. (2000) Diagnostic delay in paediatric malignancies – a population-based study. *Acta Oncology* 39, 873–6.

Timmermans, S. (1994) Dying of awareness: the theory of awareness context revisited. *Sociology of Health and Illness* 16, 322–39.

Toch, R. (1964) Management of child with a fatal disease. *Clinical Pediatrics* 3, 417–18.

Tomlinson, D. (2004) Physical restraint during procedures: issues and implications for practice. *Journal of Pediatric Oncology Nursing* 21, 258–63.

Trapani, S., Grisolia, F., Simonini, G., Calabri, G. and Falcini, F. (2000) Incidence of occult cancer in children presenting with musculoskeletal symptoms: a 10-year survey in a paediatric rheumatology unit. *Seminars in Arthritis and Rheumatology* 29, 348–59.

Tuckett, D. (1976) *An Introduction to Medical Sociology*. London: Tavistock.

Twigg, J. and Atkin, K. (1994) *Carers Perceived: Policy and Practice in Informal Care*. Buckingham: Open University Press.

Van Cleve, L., Bossert, E., Beecroft, P., Adlard., K., Alvarez, O. and Savedra, M. (2004) The pain experience of children with leukaemia during the first year after diagnosis. Nursing Research 53, 1–10.

van Dongen-Melman, J., Van Zuuren, F. and Verhulst, F. (1998) Experiences of parents of childhood cancer survivors: a qualitative analysis. *Patient Education and Counseling* 34, 185–200.

van Dulman, A. (1998) Children's contributions to pediatric outpatient encounters. *Pediatrics* 102, 563–8.

van Dulman, S. (2004) Pediatrician-parent-child communication: problem-related or not? *Patient Education and Counseling* 52, 61–8.

Vance, Y. and Eiser, C. (2004) Caring for a child with cancer – a systematic review. *Pediatric Blood Cancer* 42, 249–53.

Vance, Y. and Eiser, C. (2002) The school experience of the child with cancer. *Child: Care, Health and Development* 28, 5–19.

Vance, Y., Morse, R., Jenney, M. and Eiser, C. (2001) Issues in measuring quality of life in childhood cancer: measure, proxies and parental mental health. *Journal of Child Psychology and Psychiatry* 42, 661–7.

Vannatta, K., Garstein, M., Short, A. and Noll, R. (1998a) A controlled study of peer relationships of children surviving brain tumours: teacher, peer and self-reporting ratings. *Journal of Pediatric Psychology* 23, 279–94.

Vannatta, K., Zeller, M., Noll, R. and Koontz, K. (1998b) Social functioning of children surviving bone marrow transplantation. *Journal of Pediatric Psychology* 23, 169–78.

Varni, J., Burwinkle, T. and Katz, E. (2004) The PedsQL (tm) in pediatric cancer pain: a prospective longitudinal analysis of pain and emotional distress. *Developmental and Behavioural Pediatrics* 25, 239–46.

Varni, J., Burwinkle, T., Katz, E., Meeske, K. and Dickinson, P. (2002) The PedsQL in pediatric cancer: reliability and validity of the pediatric quality of life inventory generic core scales, multidimensional fatigue scale, and cancer module. *Cancer* 94, 2090–106.

Varni, J., Katz, E., Colegrove, R., Jr. and Dolgin, M. (1996) Family functioning predictors of adjustment of children with newly diagnosed cancer: a prospective analysis. *Journal of Child Psychology and Psychiatry* 37, 321–8.

Virtanen, R., Aromaa, M., Rautava, P., Metsahonkala, L., Anttila, P., Helenius, H. and Sillanpaa, M. (2002) Changes in headache prevalence between pre-school and pre-pubertal ages. *Cephalagia* 22, 179–85.

von Essen, L., Enskar, K., Kreuger, A., Larsson, B. and Sjoden, P. (2000) Self-esteem, depression and anxiety among young Swedish children and adolescents on and off cancer treatment. *Acta Paediatrica* 89, 229–36.

Voysey, M. (1975) *A Constant Burden: The Reconstitution of Family Life.* London: Routledge & Kegan Paul.

Wallace, W., Blacklay, A. and Eiser, C. (2001) Developing strategies for long term follow-up of survivors of childhood cancer. *British Medical Journal* 323, 271–4.

Wallander, J. and Varni, J. (1998) Effects of pediatric chronic physical disorders on child and family adjustment. *Journal of Child Psychology and Psychiatry* 39, 29–46.

Weekes, D. and Kagan, H. (1994) Adolescents completing cancer therapy: meaning, perception and coping. *Oncology Nursing Forum* 10, 663–70.

Weekes, D., Kagan, H., James, K. and Seboni, N. (1993) The phenomenon of hand holding as a coping strategy in adolescents experiencing treatment-related pain. *Journal of Pediatric Oncology Nursing* 10, 19–25.

Weigers, M., Chesler, M., Zebrack, B. and Goldman, S. (1998) Self-reported worries among long-term survivors of childhood cancer and their peers. *Journal of Psychosocial Oncology* 16, 1–23.

Wellman, H. (2002) Understanding the psychological world: developing a theory of mind, in Goswami, U., *Blackwell Handbook of Childhood Cognitive Development*, 167–87. Oxford: Blackwell Publishing.

West, P. (1990) The status and validity of accounts obtained an interview: a contrast between two studies of families with a disabled child. *Social Science and Medicine* 30, 1229–39.

Williams, C. (2000) Alert assistants in managing chronic illness: the case of mothers and teenage sons. *Sociology of Health and Illness* 22, 254–72.

Williams, C. (2002) *Mothers, Young People and Chronic Illness.* Hampshire: Ashgate.

Williams, G. (1984) The genesis of chronic illness: narrative reconstruction. *Sociology of Health and Illness* 6, 175–200.

Williams, P. (1997) Siblings and pediatric chronic illness: a review of the literature. *International Journal of Nursing Studies* 34, 312–23.

Williams, P., Williams, A., Graff, J., Hanson, S., Stanton, A., Hafeman, C., Liebergen, A., Leuenberg, K., Setter, R., Ridder, L., Curry, H., Barnard, M. and Sanders, S. (2002) Interrelationships among variables affecting well siblings and mothers in families of children with a chronic illness or disability. *Journal of Behavioural Medicine* 25, 411–424.

Williams, P., Williams, A., Graff, J., Hanson, S., Stanton, A., Hafeman, C., Lie-bergen, A., Leuenberg, K., Setter, R., Ridder, L., Curry, H., Barnard, M. and Sanders, S. (2003) A community-based intervention for siblings and parents of children with chronic illness or disability: the ISEE study. *Journal of Pediatrics* 143, 386–93.

Williams, S. and Calnan, M. (1996) *Modern Medicine: Lay Perspectives and Experiences.* London: UCL Press.

Wold, D. and Townes, B. (1969) The adjustment of siblings to childhood leukaemia. *Family Coordinator* 18, 155–60.

Wolfe, J., Klar, N., Grier, H., Duncan, J., Salem-Schatz, S., Emanuel, E. and Weeks, J. (2000) Understanding of prognosis among parents of children who died of cancer: impact on treatment goals and integration of palliative care. *JAMA* 284, 2469–75.

Woodgate, R. (2000) Part II: a critical review of qualitative research related to children's experiences with cancer. *Journal of Pediatric Oncology Nursing* 17, 207–28.

Woodgate, R. and Degner, L. (2002) 'Nothing is carved in stone': uncertainty in children with cancer and their families. *European Journal of Oncology Nursing* 6, 191–202.

Woodgate, R. and Degner, L. (2003) Expectation and beliefs about children's cancer symptoms: perspectives of children with cancer and their families. *Oncology Nursing Forum* 30, 479–91.

Woodgate, R., Degner, L. and Yanofsky, R. (2003) A different perspective to approaching cancer symptoms in children. *Journal of Pain and Symptom Management* 26, 800–17.

Woolley, H., Stein, A., Forrest, G. and Baum, J. (1989) Imparting the diagnosis of life threatening illness in children. *British Medical Journal* 298, 1623–6.

Wright, P. (1993) Parents' perceptions of their quality of life. *Journal of Pediatric Oncology Nursing* 10, 139–45.

Wyness, M. (2000) *Contesting Childhood.* London: Falmer.

Yeh, C. (2003) Dynamic coping behaviors and process of parental response to child's cancer. *Applied Nursing Research* 16, 245–55.

Yeh, C., Lin, C., Tsai, J., Lai, Y. and Ku, H. (1999) Determinants of parental decisions on 'drop out' from cancer treatment for childhood cancer patients. *Journal of Advanced Nursing* 30, 193–9.

Yeh, C., Lee, T. and Chen, M. (2000) Adaptational process of parents of pediatric oncology patients. *Pediatric Hematology and Oncology* 17, 119–31.

Young, B., Dixon-Woods, M., Findlay, M. and Heney, D. (2002) Parenting in a crisis: conceptualising mothers of children with cancer. *Social Science and Medicine* 55, 1835–47.

Young, B., Dixon-Woods, M., Windridge, K. and Heney, D. (2003) Communication with children and young people with cancer (unpublished technical report)

Young, B., Dixon-Woods, M., Windridge, K. and Heney, D. (2003) Managing communication with young people who have a potential life threatening chronic illness: qualitative study of patient and parents. *British Medical Journal* 326, 305–9.

Zebrack, B., Casillas, J., Nohr, L., Adams, H. and Zeltzer, L. (2004) Fertility issues for young adult survivors of childhood cancer. *Psycho-Oncology* 13, 689–99.

Zebrack, B. and Chesler, M. (2001) Health-related worries, self-image and life outlooks of long-term survivors of childhood cancer. *Health and Social Work* 26, 245–56.

Zebrack, B. and Chesler, M. (2002) Quality of life in childhood cancer. *Psycho-Oncology* 11, 132–41.

Zebrack, B., Chesler, M., Orbuch, T. and Parry, C. (2002a) Mothers of survivors of childhood cancer: their worries and concerns. *Journal of Psychosocial Oncology* 20, 1–25.

Zebrack, B., Zelter, L., Whitton, J., Mertens, A., Odom, L., Berkow, R. and Robison, L. (2002b) Psychological outcomes in long-term survivors of childhood leukaemia, Hodgkin's disease, and non-Hodgkin's lymphoma: a report from the childhood cancer survivor study. *Pediatrics* 110, 42–52.

Zebrack, B., Zeltzer, L., Whitton, J., Berkow, R. and Chesler, A. (2003) Survivors of childhood cancer: using siblings as a control group. *Pediatrics* 112, 1455.

Zelazo, P. and Muller, U. (2002) Executive function in typical and atypical development, in Goswami, U., *Blackwell Handbook of Childhood Cognitive Development*. 445–69. Oxford: Blackwell Publishing.

Index

This index is in word-by-word order. Page references followed by the letter 'n' indicate a reference to Notes; those in italics indicate tables and diagrams.

information about illness, 121
nausea, 53
parents response to symptoms, 38
participation in consultations, 128
psychological well-being, 56
survivors' self-assessment, 92
treatment,
    court rulings on refusal, 138, 144
    non-adherence to, 74
see also adolescence; childhood;
    children; older children

Zebrack, B.
    fertility, 118
    mental health of survivors, 83, 84
    uncertainty, 89, 106
    worries of survivors, 92
Zelazo, P., 147

GRIEF IN SCHOOL COMMUNITIES
Effective Support Strategies

Louise Rowling

This book is an essential guide for all members of a school community and other professionals who need to know how to be supportive in times of crisis - including social workers, psychologists and bereavement specialists. Whilst the emphasis of many books about young people and loss and grief has been on how to support those young people as individuals in a family context, this book takes a different approach and uses 'the school community' as the organizing supportive framework. This approach recognises that losses are embedded in a young person's social environment - the school and its community, as well as the family. The theoretical orientation utilised is that death and all loss experiences are interpreted through social interaction and experienced within a social context.

The book is firmly based on theory, research and practice. It breaks new ground in demonstrating the components in a school that can be used to support grieving individuals in times of personal crisis and to support whole school communities when traumatic incidents occur. Within this comprehensive approach attention is given to the needs and experiences of personnel - teachers, students, school leaders, parents; as well as school policies and programs and links with outside services.

Contents: *Foreword – Preface – Acknowledgements – Frameworks for a comprehensive approach to loss and grief in schools – Impact of loss on children and adolescents – Teachers being human – Grief and the classroom – Critical incident management – Supportive school environment – Being in charge – Grief and family/school relationships – Partnerships with outside agencies – Special cases – Disenfranchised grief in schools – Education and training – References – Index.*

208pp 0 335 21115 1 (Paperback)

CANCER IN YOUNG ADULTS
Through Parents' Eyes

Anne Grinyer

The original inspiration for this book was George, who died from osteosarcoma at the age of 23. During his illness his parents tried, without success, to access information on the life-stage issues that make life-threatening illness during young adulthood particularly difficult to manage. They could find no literature relating specifically to this problem and struggled throughout George's 4 years of living with cancer to cope with the additional problems faced by families in this situation. After his death they set up a research project to help other families facing these issues. This book is the outcome of that research. It is heavily based on the use of narrative material written by parents whose young adult children have been diagnosed with cancer.

The book addresses issues such as sexuality and fertility, independence, the need for normality, the effect on siblings, the ownership of medical information, financial issues, the impact on the parents' partnership and the emotional consequences of the illness. It is designed to be of practical assistance both to parents and to health professionals involved with the care of young adults with cancer.

Contents: Series editor's preface – Acknowledgements – Foreword written by George's mother Helen – The impact of illness on family life – The loss of independence: the impact on family dynamics – Seeking 'normality' – Sexuality and fertility: confronting the 'taboo' – Involvement in medical decisions: who owns the knowledge? – The effect on siblings: managing conflicting demands – The financial implications for the family – Effects on marital relationships – The emotional challenge – A reflection on the book: its purpose, process and ethics – Biographies – Appendix: Examples of the calls for narratives – Bibliography – Index.

208pp 0 335 21230 1 (Paperback) 0 335 21231 X (Hardback)

LOSS, CHANGE AND BEREAVEMENT IN PALLIATIVE CARE

Pam Firth, Gill Luff and David Oliviere

- How do professionals meet the needs of bereaved people?
- How do professionals undertake best practice with individuals, groups, families and communities?
- What are the implications for employing research to influence practice?

This book provides a resource for working with a complex range of loss situations and includes chapters on childhood bereavement, and individual and family responses to loss and change. It contains the most up-to-date work in the field presented by experienced practitioners and researchers and is relevant not only for those working in specialist palliative care settings, but for professionals in general health and social care sectors.

Strong links are maintained between research and good practice throughout the book. These are reinforced by the coherent integration of international research material and the latest thinking about loss and bereavement. Experts and clinicians draw upon their knowledge and practice, whilst the essential perspective of the service user is central to this book.

Loss, Change and Bereavement in Palliative Care provides essential reading for a range of professional health and social care disciplines practising at postgraduate or post-registration/qualification level. It challenges readers, at an advanced level, on issues of loss, change and bereavement.

Contributors:
Lesley Adshead, Jenny Altschuler, Peter Beresford, Grace H. Christ, Suzy Croft, Pam Firth, Shirley Firth, Richard Harding, Felicity Hearn, Jennie Lester, Gill Luff, Linda Machin, Jan McLaren, David Oliviere, Ann Quinn, Phyllis R. Silverman, Jean Walker, Karen Wilman.

Contents: *Notes on the contributors – Series editor's preface – Acknowledgements – Foreword – Introduction – The context of loss, change and bereavement in palliative care – Mourning: a changing view – Research in practice – Illness and loss within the family – Life review with the terminally ill – narrative therapies – The death of a child – Interventions with bereaved children – Involving service users in palliative care: from theory to practice – Excluded and vulnerable groups of service users – Carers: current research and developments – Groupwork in palliative care – Cultural perspectives on loss and bereavement – Conclusions – Index.*

240pp   0 335 21323 5 (Paperback)   0 335 21324 3 (Hardback)

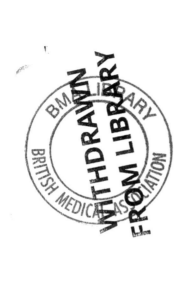

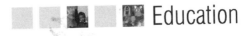
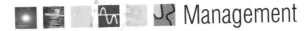
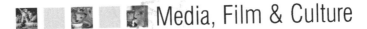
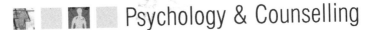
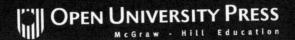